BEASTLY BODY

THE ESSENTIAL GUIDE TO BICEPS, CALVES, AND GLUTES GROWTH AND DEVELOPMENT

RHYS LARSON

CONTENTS

KILLER CALVES

BEASTLY BICEPS

GLORIOUS GLUTES

KILLER CALVES

THE ESSENTIAL GUIDE TO CALF GROWTH AND DEVELOPMENT

RHYS LARSON

PREFACE

A few words of caution and encouragement.

This book is about helping you reach your potential, and getting your calves to grow.

Although pushing your limits helps you—and your calves—grow and improve, you should exercise thoughtfully and with common sense.

As you work to build your calves, don't take unnecessary risks or push yourself too hard, especially not to the point of injury.

Please consult a physician before embarking on any exercise program, especially if you have any questions or concerns about your body, your health, or your exercise limitations, and please do not do these exercises except under medical guidance if you usually don't specifically exercise your calves at all.

I want you **healthy** and exercising, rather than injured and exercising or not exercising at all!

It's the only way for those stubborn calves to actually benefit and grow.

—Rhys Larson

KILLER CALVES

Not everyone is born with the calves of their dreams. Whether you want calves that are well-formed, defined, supple, huge, or ripped, *Killer Calves* can help make your dreams a reality.

For those who want to banish their chicken legs to the distant past, *Killer Calves* will help turn your shrimpy calves into raging bulls.

If you want to be fit, bring variety to your exercise routines, add some lower leg development, or maintain what you have already worked so hard to attain, *Killer Calves* is for you too.

Killer Calves offers a wide range of tools, exercises, insights, and ideas to help shape your legs, particularly your calves.

So, if you're a hard gainer who has tried everything—or think you have —to build your calves, *Killer Calves* will give you numerous new ways to push your limits and help your muscles grow. If you're looking to sculpt and tone your lower legs, *Killer Calves* will provide you with a host of options to achieve the look you're after. Or, if you're already jacked and looking to add a bit of variety and new options to your leg routine, *Killer Calves* will give you novel ideas and programs to torture yourself at home and the gym.

Whether you're a fitness beginner looking for help, a seasoned bodybuilder or fitness professional looking for that little edge, someone who wants to get in shape, or an exercise enthusiast looking for a new approach, *Killer Calves* will help you improve your legs.

Everyone deserves a great pair of legs.

Everyone deserves a pair of killer calves!

HOW THIS BOOK WORKS

Killer Calves has been devised around the idea of giving you all the necessary knowledge and tools to get your calves to grow and develop the way you'd like them to.

To do this, *Killer Calves* is broken into sections that will give you numerous tips and exercise routines to try out. The options include basic exercises you may already know to off-the-wall ideas you've never heard of, much less tried.

These routines can be performed on their own or combined with other exercise programs. Added into your leg days, the exercises detailed here in *Killer Calves* will deliver so much more of an impact and intensity than just your standard calf circuit.

More than just your regular exercises and routines, *Killer Calves* will also provide you with differing techniques and variations for each exercise. These aim toward maximizing growth and training effectiveness, simultaneously delivering useful background information on basic anatomy and how the calves function, helping you understand how to best achieve the calf development you're seeking.

Finally—and this is a major inspiration for writing *Killer Calves*—by bringing all these ideas and approaches together in one place, I hope it will inspire you to experiment, explore, and learn which approaches work best for you. By learning techniques you'll love and value, I hope you will share how to get killer calves with anyone who's needing a boost to their leg game or struggling to meet their fitness goals.

Remember, the end goal of the calf development odyssey is yours to choose—whether it's colossal calves or simply sleek, defined, well-proportioned legs. Whatever outcome you decide, *Killer Calves* is here to make those goals possible.

CALFCENTRIC DEDICATION

Don't let anyone tell you that training your calves is easy. More than most other body parts, getting your calves to grow can be demanding, frustrating, and taxing. For some, the quest for calf development can even become all-consuming.

And, like almost anything worthwhile, getting the calves of your dreams requires dedication and hard work.

Lots of it.

This process is also not simple or quick, so if you came here hoping to land on a quick fix for your chicken legs, you're going to be disappointed. But don't give up!

Killer Calves will give you tools to help your calves grow through numerous ways to attack your weakest link and stimulate improvement.

But as with anything else worthwhile, you have to be dedicated to bring about change. You have to be committed and put forth the necessary effort.

Simply reading and understanding a workout, or going through the motions as you exercise will not get you where you want to be. Just signing up to the gym with a view to putting these exercises through their paces won't do a thing for you if you never attend and put yourself through the recommended exercises—and often.

Realize in the first place that your calves are used and worked every day, and so are resilient and resistant to change. To overcome this challenge, you have to be just as dedicated and determined as your calves are stubborn and reluctant. Essentially, you're going head to head with your stubborn calves and not taking no for an answer!

You have to counter their resistance to growth, and believe me, they will seem to throw out plenty of excuses along the way. But again, no amount of knowledge or range of exercises will do anything for you *if you don't make them count.*

And you are the only one who can do that for yourself.

Killer Calves will get you started on your way to the legs of your dreams, *but you are the one who has to get there...* one calf raise at a time.

Just in case you chose not to read the above, let's say again:

You are the one who has to get there. Nobody else can do it for you.

Train diligently, persevere, and embody your end goals with every repetition. Push yourself to reach your dreams because no one else will do it for you.

And then you, too, will have killer calves.

CALF PRIORITIZATION

Not only does training your calves require "calfcentric" focus and attention, but also, developing your calves requires prioritization. If you want to turn a weakness into a strength, you have to devote yourself to change, working creatively and strategically toward turning your liability into an asset, and putting forth the effort and dedication to see your goals through.

If calves are your weakness, you have to make them a priority.

It's that simple.

Think of the problem of helping your calves grow and develop in terms of common workout programs and goals... normal fitness frameworks and paradigms. People go to the gym all the time, primarily for their chest days, back days, and arm days.

But how often do people go to the gym for calf days?

Even on leg days, calves are often an afterthought if they're worked at all, and far too often neglected.

When your gym buddies are bragging about their latest workout or new routine, chances are they are not talking about their calves or everything they did on calf day. There are so many articles in books, magazines, and online, focusing on every single other body part... except calf day.

Sure, there are articles on calf exercises and programs, but the calves are generally treated as a secondary muscle group to be incorporated into a leg workout or as an afterthought.

With *Killer Calves*, I'm here to change that.

Together, we're going to make calves a priority.

We're going to make every day calf day!

CALF EXERCISE OVERVIEW

Before diving into the exercises, programs, and concepts presented in *Killer Calves*, here's a brief overview of the exercise types you'll use to add life, definition, and volume to your calves. Since there are so many specific calf exercises I'll be using in this book, I've broken these down into the general body position needed when performing the necessary exercise movements. This way, when discussing exercises and routines in more detail, you'll have an idea of what's expected and how to get started.

1. **Standing calf exercises** – Standing calf exercises are calf raises performed in a standing position—on or off a machine, on one leg or two, and with or without weights. At the gym, do these exercises on a standing calf-raise machine, on a squat rack or Smith machine, with dumbbells or kettlebells, or on one leg or two. At home, you may or may not have similar equipment as at the gym, but you can still perform standing calf exercises with or without weights, on the stairs, on steps, on the floor, or any elevated ledge that will support your weight. I'll discuss the many variations you can add throughout the rest of the book, to help you get the most out of your calf program.

2. **Seated calf exercises** – Seated calf raises are performed, as the name rightly suggests, while you are seated, generally using some form of equipment. Seated calf exercises can be performed with legs straight—on a leg press machine, or with legs bent—as with a seated calf machine. At the gym, seated calf exercises are generally performed with legs straight on a leg-press machine as an alternative or supplement to standing calf exercises because they also hit the gastrocnemius muscles. Seated calf exercises are performed on the seated calf machine with bent legs, with the exertion focusing on the soleus muscles. At home, assuming you don't have a leg press or seated calf-raise machine, seated calf exercises can be performed using a chair, with your legs bent and with weights resting on your knees and thighs, or while squatting with knees bent completely to mimic the seated calf-raise machine. Whether your legs are straight or bent, your calf exercises can be performed on one or two legs depending on how much weight or intensity you need. Almost any variation used with standing calf raises can be performed with seated calf raises.

3. **Calf exercises with a bent waist** – Calf exercises with a bent waist are generally performed either seated at the leg-press machine or standing with a bent waist for donkey calf raises. With seated calf raises on the leg press, the weight rests on your feet. In contrast, with donkey calf raises—performed standing with a bent waist—the weight rests on your waist or lower back. Donkey calf raises can be performed on a donkey calf-raise machine, with weights hanging from around your waist, or with partners sitting on your lower back. At home, you will need to be creative to perform donkey calf raises and other standing bent waist calf exercise variations but suspending a weight from your waist will work if no family or friends volunteer to help.

4. **Dynamic calf exercises** – Although your body is moving during the other calf exercise positions, you are generally holding most of your body static through the exercises to focus the primary exertion within your calves. In contrast, dynamic calf exercises tend to be explosive and plyometric in nature, involving more of

your body as you lift, jump, and exert powerfully, often leaving the ground as you thrust up or ahead. Jumping and sprinting exercises are typically the focus of dynamic calf exercises and range from jumping rope or jumping vertically in place, to plyometric leaps and hill sprints.

Although I've given a rough overview of calf-raise exercise types and the positions used in each category, there are many variations and options to add variety and intensity to these techniques. As you read, explore, and undertake your personal calf development journey, together we'll build on these foundational exercises throughout *Killer Calves*. The better your foundation, the better your calves.

EXERCISE VARIATIONS

Killer Calves is filled with different exercises and approaches to develop your calves. But one thing I need to stress is that you will ultimately have to find out what works best to achieve your calf goals. Whatever exercises and techniques you try, you will need to be persistent, maximize your effort, listen to your body, and, above all else, be willing to push your boundaries to achieve your dreams.

Every exercise routine in *Killer Calves* can be modified and adapted to help you grow and push your limits. Think of yourself as a mad fitness scientist searching out the best ways to unlock your growth potential. This process takes some work and quite a bit of creativity. Use this opportunity, your focused effort, and your ingenuity to your advantage to help yourself grow!

So, as you try out the routines and ideas in *Killer Calves*, here are some variations for almost any exercise to push your limits, overcome boredom and muscle adaptation, and build those calves! Ways to vary almost any exercise include:

1. **Reps** – Vary the number of repetitions required to push your limits. As your strength and endurance grow, increase the

weight you push and/or the number of repetitions you perform.

2. **Sets** – Like reps, increasing or decreasing the numbers of sets by exercise type is always an option for calf development, whether your focus is on mass or definition.

3. **Time under tension** – Vary the time working, the time spent moving through the exercise, the time held contracting the calf at the top of the raise, and the time relaxed at the bottom of the motion to reduce or extend the time of your physical exertion.

4. **Weight** – Adding or subtracting weight is one of the classic ways to vary exercises. Not only can you add or subtract weight as you work through your sets, but you can also do the same within a set—drop sets or reverse drop sets. This will allow you to not only increase your total load—the amount of weight lifted in a given set—but can also extend your time under tension as you fight against muscle failure, such as when performing drop sets, to facilitate muscle growth.

5. **Explosivity** – Adjust the amount of energy or plyometric activation in each exercise. For instance, explode up during the calf raise and then lower slowly, or accelerate through your lift starting slowly and gradually building speed as you elevate.

6. **Change how you move through the exercise** – Employ continuous and discontinuous movements to shock your calves. For example, include pulses at the top of your calf raise while holding at full muscle extension and muscular concentration or include pauses or holds mid-motion.

7. **Exercise orientation** – Shift your foot orientation during the exercise. Classic examples include moving your toes out, pointing your toes in, or directing your toes forward during exercise.

8. **Change stress and strain direction** – Shift where the exercise tension moves through your calves by changing where the exertion moves through your feet when you push upward. For example, pushing up from and through your big toes instead of lifting from the balls of your feet or outside of them.

9. **Adjust the orientation of your bodyweight** – During exercise,

adjust your body's angle to shift how the weight and exercise tension move through your muscles. For instance, lean forward, backward, sideways, or stay centered during the exercise to increase intensity and alter the focus of exertion.

10. **Adjust the smoothness or continuity of your motions** – Although you'll naturally tend to move fluidly through an exercise with continuity of motion, changing this will shock your muscles. Instead of completing the whole movement in one smooth motion, break it into sections.

11. **Surprise to overcome adaptation** – Change your routines to continue pushing your development. If your calves have adapted to your routine, their growth will suffer. A simple way to evaluate this is if they are no longer sore the day after your workout. If your calves aren't sore, consider changing your routine or increasing your workout intensity. If you haven't shocked your calves to the point of soreness, they are not going to respond with much growth.

12. **Electrical Muscle Stimulation (EMS)** – Stimulating your muscles with electrical impulses can certainly shock them into growth. Some muscles respond more effectively than others to EMS training. In the case of calves, using EMS stimulation during your exercise routine, specifically in conjunction with weights and intense exertion, not only offers a novel way to train but can speed up results. In this instance, EMS can simulate adding additional weight and intensity to your calf routine without the risks of additional weight such as muscle tears, tendon damage, and joint pain. Consider EMS as another option to push yourself in new and growth-inducing ways.

13. **Combinations** – Any of these variations can be combined to add variety and increase effectiveness to your calf exercises, and, finally,

14. **Be original** – Think of your own variations to add to the list.

Variety is not only the spice of life; it is a key component of calf growth. Use these variations to keep your routines fresh and your calves growing!

Remember, this is a book about calf-building. So, although you often need to push your limits to get your calves to grow, you also need to be able to use them. Exercise intelligently and listen to your body to avoid injury. If you push yourself too hard, to the point of injury or inability to work out regularly, you won't be able to work those calves and your goals will suffer. Being out of action due to injury or discomfort for a few days is not going to help your calf growth goals, so take it steady and at an appropriate pace.

WAYS TO INCREASE YOUR CALVES' ABILITY TO GROW AND IMPROVE

Calves are stubborn. More than almost any other muscle group, they seem resistant to growth. To get your calves to respond, you need to find ways to overcome this resistance and increase their ability to respond to training.

Several factors can reduce or strongly influence your calves' potential to improve:

1. Your calves are highly adaptable muscles since you use them daily, even when not formally training.
2. Your calf anatomy—the attachment points of your calf muscle fibers on each leg, such as high versus low insertion points. High calf insertions reduce the overall growth area for the calf muscle while low calf insertions increase this area.
3. Failure to use proper form during exercise. Examples of improper form include using a short range of motion and bouncing without proper muscle control through the movement. Improper form reduces time under tension, limiting muscle fiber engagement and growth potential.
4. Your calves have a very high elasticity or ability to stretch and rebound during exertion, allowing the calf muscle to extend

more than two thirds of its range of motion and then recover
quickly from tension transfer mediated by the Achilles tendon.

5. Your calf muscles' ratio of muscle fiber types—the percentage of
   fast versus slow twitch muscle fibers.

To maximize your growth potential, you need to attack and overcome the
limiting factors you *can* control—your range of motion, muscle engagement, and time under tension.

To maximize your growth potential, for every repetition, increase the
time under tension, maximize muscle engagement and exertion, put your
awareness and focus into the muscle, and work to reduce the role of
Achilles tendon elasticity during exercise—since the Achilles tendon
reduces the calf muscles' contribution during each movement.

Combined, these approaches will ensure that the calf muscles do the
majority of the work as you exercise. This means no bouncing, no partial
reps, no releasing muscular tension, and no slacking... at least not until
you've reached a point where you can't do much else or where exercises
call for different techniques!

To help overcome these limitations, every single rep should be done
with good form. Here's how. Consider this the foundational calf-raise form
on which you'll build as your strength and experience grow:

1. Hold the stretch position—the lowest, fully extended position in
   most calf exercises—for at least two seconds to counter tendon
   elasticity, i.e. the Achilles tendon's capacity to stretch, transfer
   energy, and reduce full muscle engagement. Try to maintain
   tension in your hold—the stretch position is not a passive stretch
   and, to the extent possible, your muscles should be engaged.

2. Move slowly through the entire range of motion, especially the
   beginning of the reps, with control. Avoid accelerating and
   bouncing, so that you are controlling the weight and moving
   with purpose.

3. Hold the topmost contracted position—the highest, fully

extended position in most calf exercises—for at least two seconds. Squeeze the muscle hard and put your mind—and your attention—into the muscle as you work.

4. Maintain maximum muscle tension as you lower the weight down. Resist the weight while you perform a controlled, negative exertion. You do not drop the weight down—you lower it through its full motion.

Calf growth routine:

Perform this superset to help boost your calf growth:

1. **Seated Calf Raises** – Using the principles of good form outlined above, perform 10-12 reps with no rest.
2. **Sled Pushing** – with a heavy load, push a weighted sled for 30 seconds.
3. **Rest** for 2 minutes. For best results, repeat the superset 2 to 3 more times.

With slow, controlled sets using maximal stretch and extension, full muscle engagement, and proper attention, your calves' ability to respond to training may surprise you.

BE THE CALF

Do your calves make chopsticks look thick?

The right program and frame of mind can fix that.

All you have to do is put your mind to it.

The secret to building phenomenal calves isn't about how much weight you can get them to move, although heavy weights *can* help. The secret to great calves is *being the calf*, feeling the calf muscles work through the entire range of exertion. Put your mind inside your muscles as you contract and relax.

Put your awareness in the muscles *throughout* your exercises.

But you're not just watching; you're engaging. This attention gets you to work, not watch. Use your awareness to enlist more muscle fibers, to stimulate the right muscles, to correct improper form, and to push harder and more completely than you would just counting reps or holding a position for some time.

Fully engaging in your exercises will not only focus your attention, but it will also stimulate your muscles through greater activation, help you observe opportunities for improvement, and spur your muscles on to greater growth.

Calves are no exception.

. . .

Use the following techniques to build your mind-muscle connection and encourage calf growth:

Seated Calf Flexes – Sit in a chair with your feet flat on the ground and legs bent at a 90-degree angle. Maintaining the seated, bent-legged position, lift up onto your toes one leg at a time. Hold this elevated position with your feet at full extension for 10 seconds. Contract your muscles, flexing as hard as you can while supporting your leg weight, then lower the foot and repeat, performing 3 to 4 calf flexes per side. The more seated calf flexes you perform each day, the better results you'll have.

Align Your Hips Properly – The angle of your hips plays a significant role in where you target your calf muscles, e.g., in the medial vs. lateral head muscles of the gastrocnemius. Involve the internal vs. external rotation angle of your hips in your calf training to find an angle that creates maximum calf muscle burn. Use the following steps to help adjust your hip alignment for targeted calf growth:

1. Start with your feet in a regular shoulder-width stance.
2. To focus on external hip rotation, keep your heels on the ground and rotate your toes away from one another, so that your heels are roughly shoulder-width apart while your toes shift out.
3. To focus on internal hip rotation, keep your toes on the ground and rotate your heels away from one another, so that your toes are roughly shoulder-width apart while your heels shift out.
4. For many people, the optimal angle will be about 45-degrees, but you will need to experiment to find what works best for you. Remember, you are looking for the angle that creates the most muscle burn. When performing targeted calf raises, do all your sets and reps at that angle.

Stand and Flex – Whenever you're standing in one place for extended periods, push up onto your toes using both calves, and flex. Hold this position until your calves start shaking, performing an extended isometric calf contraction. This isometric hold is perfect for when you're standing at your desk, standing by your counter cooking, working at a benchtop, or performing any other activity that gives the opportunity to carry out the exercise. Standing and flexing in place is also a great way to boost the mind-muscle connection with your calves—and your gains!

Every day is calf day – I mean it! Every time you work out, perform one set of calf exercises. Do this set on any suitable equipment using any calf-focused exercise, such as a standing calf-raise machine, a leg press, a seated calf-raise machine, a squat rack, or a donkey calf-raise machine. After warming up, do one pyramid set as below:

1. Using your chosen exercise, perform 10 reps using a full range of motion. Go as high onto your toes as you possibly can on the last rep. Don't come down onto your heels after the last rep. Instead, do a 10-second isolation hold. Just hold that contraction at the top and squeeze hard. Put your mind—and effort—into the muscle.
2. Without rest, do another 10 reps. Go back into another 10-second isolation hold at full extension on the tips of your toes. As you fatigue, these may turn into partial reps. Fatigue and failure are okay; just don't give up.
3. Finally, to completely burn out your muscles, do another round of 10 reps and finish with one last 10-second isolation hold, going up onto your toes as high as possible. If your calves are not on fire and you can still perform complete reps by this point, you need to add more weight.
4. To help with recovery, immediately after the final isometric hold, lower your calves all the way down, and let the weight push down through your calves to stretch them. Hold this stretch for as long as possible. Alternate legs on the stretch as needed.
5. For the first week, do this program once per workout. After the

first week, try to go through the workout twice. You might find it difficult to walk but your calves will grow.

The mind-muscle connection is exceptionally important for muscle growth. The mind-body connection, particularly learning to use this effectively, is also one of the weakest links in most people's overall fitness. Strengthen the mind-body link and your calves will have a shot at becoming the ideal you dream of every day.

TRAIN YOUR CALVES WITH STRAIGHT LEGS—A LITTLE CALF ANATOMY TO HELP YOUR MUSCLES GROW

Yes, your calves are stubborn, but, with a little understanding of *why* your calves aren't growing, you'll finally make them grow.

Your calves are comprised of three distinct muscle heads, the medial and lateral gastrocnemius, along with the underlying soleus.

While all three muscles have a distal attachment to the Achilles tendon that inserts onto the back of the heel, the proximal attachments are what separates the true calf muscles—the gastrocnemius—from the soleus.

The gastrocnemius are considered "dual joint" muscles because they cross two joints—the ankle and the knee. Most people don't understand this point, utilize this information, or effectively incorporate this understanding into their training.

In contrast to the gastrocnemius, the soleus muscle attaches onto the back side of the lower leg bones and never crosses the knee joint.

The soleus muscle only crosses the ankle joint.

This anatomical differentiation between the gastrocnemius and soleus muscles plays a major role in preventing people from building and developing their calf muscles.

Why does this anatomical difference matter?

Many people end up performing the calf raise movement incorrectly… at least for ideal muscle growth. Instead of stressing the gastrocnemius muscles, their training targets the stabilizer muscles of the lower leg, known as the soleus and medial flexor group.

With poor form, they miss out on fully engaging the two primary muscles in the calf that you want to grow to be aesthetically pleasing—to be ripped, full, huge, defined, or proportional to the rest of your body—the gastrocnemius.

To most effectively hit the gastrocnemius, ensure the knee is placed in a fully extended—straight—position when doing standing calf raises. The gastrocnemius muscles pass the knee joint and play a role in slight knee flexion. They also stabilize the knee. So, with this understanding in mind, the gastrocnemius *must* be trained with a straight-knee position to fully engage the calf muscles.

Most chicken-legged gym-goers do standing calf raises with slightly bent knees which shifts the emphasis to the soleus and flexors and else-where in the body, taking the weight away from the gastrocnemius.

So, the next time you're doing calf raises, especially while standing, use a full range of motion and make sure you maintain straight knees throughout the set.

You'll instantly feel the difference.

And your calves will thank you.

SLOW DOWN TO SPEED UP GAINS

Have you already tried standing calf raises with little success?

If so, you may be doing them incorrectly.

Your calves' weakness might come from one of your body's greatest strengths, your Achilles tendon, the thickest tendon in the body. The Achilles is meant for dynamic and explosive movements. So, whenever you hop on a standing calf-raise machine and bounce up and down banging out reps, your Achilles tendons have no problems managing that work, relieving the tension—and the workload—from the calves.

So, to see any gains, you have to target and isolate your calves during the workout.

To shift that work from the Achilles to the calves, you need to slow down and stop. Doing this as you perform your reps will remove as much of the Achilles' elastic stretch rebound as possible and focus on maximally lengthening and shortening your calf muscles. Slow down through the movement, pausing while fully extended for most benefit. Combining this controlled movement with straight legs—in standing calf raises—will also prevent the tension from moving away from the gastrocnemius and into other leg areas.

Here's how to perform calf raises with a minimum 8-second pause in your reps to unlock their growth potential:

1. Hold the stretch position—the bottom position of your calf raises with your heels lowered as much as possible—for 5 seconds on every rep.
2. With your knees straight—to keep the tension on your calves and not elsewhere in your legs—push up slowly, controlling the weight with your exertion.
3. Hold the contracted position—the top position at full extension —for at least 3 seconds on every rep.
4. Lower slowly, engaging your muscles as you drop, then repeat.
5. Perform 4 sets of 12 reps in each set, rotating through different calf exercise variations each time you work them, such as changing toe positions.
6. Carry out this calf routine at least twice a week. As you get stronger, add more weight and/or increase the time taken for each repetition of the calf raise. You could also hold your contractions and stretches for longer.

If you've been bouncing when working your calves, then the difference in feeling your muscles actually work will be striking. Also, because you'll be working your calves instead of your tendons, be prepared for more muscle soreness. As an added bonus, the extended time held in the stretch position during calf raises will also help to stretch out your Achilles tendons if they're tight.

And remember, when training your calves, slow, controlled motions speed up gains.

VARIETY IS THE SPICE OF LIFE...FOR CALF GAINS

Don't blame your genetics for your weak lower legs. Blame your training —or its absence. Many weightlifters' calf workouts involve rapid, shallow reps... that's if they do any training for calves at all, of course.

When you exercise, don't be a calf bouncer or bobber. Getting your calves to grow requires loaded flexion and extension of the ankles. Most people neglect this important point and miss a significant side benefit of calf training: strong feet and ankles.

Poor exercise mechanics doesn't just hurt your calf gains though.

Poor mechanics when exercising your calves ultimately affects your gains and performance of other important lifts too.

Here are some tools to strengthen your feet, improve your ankle mobility, help your calves grow bigger, and improve the entire foundation of your lower-body training to help you squat, deadlift, press, and grow with the best of them.

Paused Calf Raises - If you are like most gym goers, you've probably been doing calf raises as though you're bouncing on a trampoline. While this may make you think you're working out your calves as you throw around heavy weights, you're really just putting your Achilles tendons through their paces. Don't fool yourself. Bouncy, shallow reps are not the way to get your calves to grow.

Athletes depend on the elastic nature of the Achilles tendon for jumping, running, and rapid movement shifts. But Achilles training will not build your calves. Look no further than the kangaroo. What has elastic bouncing done for kangaroos' calves? If you want kangaroo calves, however, bounce away.

If you allow elastic, springy movements to predominate in your calf training, you'll reduce the effectiveness of your calf exercises. Pausing at the top and bottom on any calf raise will limit the Achilles tendon's involvement in the exercise. Without this elastic contribution, your calf muscles will do more work. More work equals more growth. More control equals less Achilles involvement.

When performing your calf raises, pause at the top and bottom of the motion for at least two seconds. Stretch the calf at the bottom as much as possible without pain by allowing your heels to drop and your toes to point upward. Then, after this pause, push as high as possible onto the balls of your feet and toes. Hold your calf raise again at the top of the lift.

If you want to develop better strength and mobility at the end of your exertion ranges in your calf exercises—under full downward stretch and upward contraction in the hold positions at the top and bottom of the rep —you should work on controlling the exercise movements under load at the tops and bottoms of your lifts. As you gain more control in the tops and bottoms of your lifts, your ankles and feet will grow stronger. Take a similar approach to reap benefits in other exercises as well, such as squatting, benching, curls, or any other exercise.

To start, choose a load you're able to control and press with full ankle dorsiflexion and extension or you'll default to bouncing the weight. Allow yourself to settle into the stretch using the weight as a guide. Use a similar approach to your other calf-raise variations.

If your calves are tight and prevent you getting a full stretch at the bottom of your exercise, then try foam rolling to release the muscles. Alternate between foam rolling your calves for 10 rolls and static stretching them for 20-30 seconds each. Repeat 2 to 3 times and then try flexing your ankles. Be persistent and keep stretching over time to help get your flexibility where it's needed. If you have damaged your ankles from past injuries and have ankle sprains and strains, for example, then stretching becomes very important to overcome potential movement limitations.

Also, be sure to vary your rep ranges and train your calves frequently. Our calves evolved to let us stand and walk on them all day and each day. Doing 3 to 4 sets of 8-10 reps once a week won't shock your muscle into growth.

Tiptoe Farmer's Carries - Farmers, used to physical labor, are often far stronger than you might guess, especially based on appearances. Hauling around heavy objects such as sacks of feed, machine parts, and other necessities daily is part of the reason they're so strong. Use the farmer's secret weapon—lifting heavy stuff as you move—as a key to calf development.

To get started, pick up suitable weights—the heavier the better—and walk on your tiptoes across the gym, your living room, or wherever you're working out. Don't worry about any strange looks you may receive as you move around; those looks will turn to envy as your calves grow. Channel your inner farmer or strongman as you lug around those dumbbells. Use the tiptoe farmer carry as a more effective alternative to the seated calf machine.

Tip: Use a weight that allows you to maintain full ankle plantar flexion —a full extension onto the balls of your feet, extending up onto your tiptoes as you stand. This will strengthen your feet, help develop ankle control, and smash your calves.

Single-Leg Kettlebell Passes - One of the most effective ways to strengthen your ankles, feet, and calves is to do challenging single-leg exercises. Examples include single-leg squats, split-squat variations, and single-leg deadlifts. As you balance on them, the muscles in your feet and ankles work harder because you engage stability muscles. This balancing act also makes you focus your attention on the muscles working to keep you stable, creating a forced mind-muscle connection. Stronger feet and ankles play a key role in your ability to handle heavier weights and in getting your calves to grow.

Challenge your arches and ankles with this simple drill. Stronger arches and ankles are especially valuable for those who overpronate or have flat feet.

Stand on one leg holding a kettlebell in one hand at your side. While maintaining balance on one foot, slowly pass the kettlebell across your body and over to the opposing hand. You can also perform this exercise with a dumbbell, but, given its ergonomics, a kettlebell is easier to pass between hands. Slowly pass the kettlebell to the opposite hip, hold for a moment, and then reverse the movement. Pass the kettlebell back and forth for 4 to 6 passes for 2 to 3 sets on each leg. Progressive loading matters less than maintaining control and balance in the exercise.

Sled Pushes - Many people think of sleds as a tool for conditioning, athletic training, or for hauling presents at Christmas. But the sled also works for those seeking bigger, stronger physiques—especially calves and legs—and a better overall work capacity.

Sled pushing is concentric-focused, so the exercise doesn't cause serious soreness like some other calf exercises. Sled pushing is a safe, effective way to load and train your calves and ankles in the way they're meant to move. To top off your overall gains, sled pushing engages your glutes and quads in addition to your calves, adding a variety of benefits to your routine.

As you perform the exercise, take natural, deliberate strides while you push a loaded sled over 20 to 50 yards or meters of turf. Maintain tension in your abdominal muscles for stability and keep a natural, neutral spine as you move your hips with each stride. As you work, use the ground to push the sled forward, connecting solidly through your feet. Load the sled with additional weight to do some serious exercise.

Perform 3 to 4 sets of sled pushes after any workout for some high-intensity anaerobic interval training.

Calf training doesn't have to be a chore.

Use the exercises in *Killer Calves* to not only improve your calf development and overcome plateaus but to keep your workouts fun and enjoyable.

Remember, the more you enjoy your workouts, the more likely you are to do them on a regular basis. And regular, dedicated exercise is a vital key to calf growth.

CALF ROUTINES OF THE HUGE AND FAMOUS

Many people are famous for their physiques, just as there are many who are famous for their knowledge. There are also some who are famous for their calves.

Here, I'll spread a bit of these calf legends' knowledge so that you can enjoy their phenomenal physiques.

Arnold Schwarzenegger's Conan Calves[1]

Arnold is a true legend, and so are his calves. Arnold, among many other things, is famous for transforming his calves from tiny saplings into mighty oaks.

Here are a couple of Arnold's routines:

Arnold's Calf Routine 1:

Exercise	Sets	Reps
Monday / Wednesday / Friday		
Donkey Calf Raises	4	10
Standing Calf Raises	4	10
Seated Calf Raises	4	10
Tuesday / Thursday / Saturday		
Standing Calf Raises	4	15, 10, 8, 8
Calf Raises on a Leg-Press Machine	4	10

Arnold believes in the benefits of volume training with high training loads to stimulate muscle growth, and this routine reflects these volume-based beliefs. This program also shows how much Arnold believes in and dedicates to working his calves. This routine requires being totally committed to your calf development, and in the gym six days a week. As in many of Arnold's routines, his programs are a gold standard of fitness—well thought out, proven, comprehensive, and results-driven.

Arnold's Calf Routine 2:

Donkey Calf Raise - Sets: 5-6, Reps: 15-20.
Standing Calf Raise - Sets: 5-6, Reps: 10-20.
Seated Calf Raise - Sets: 4-5, Reps: 10-15.

Arnold's advice on calf training in his own words:

"The main exercises I did shouldn't surprise you: donkey calf raises, standing calf raises, seated calf raises, and leg press calf raises—up to six sets of each for 10–20 reps. But more important than the exercise I was doing, or the number of sets and reps I performed, was how I did them.

"To develop your calves to their potential, you must take each rep through a complete range of motion. This means getting a full stretch at the bottom and forcing yourself up as high as possible on your toes at the top.

Again, it's about progression; if you're using 1,000 pounds but can't go all the way up, you're training too heavy and wasting your time. The goal is to lift the heaviest weight possible that still allows you to use a full range of motion.

"I also used other techniques to squeeze out every last bit of intensity and spark new growth. Other than doing forced reps with the help of a partner, my favorite techniques were peak contractions and what I used to call a 'pumping action'.

"Peak contraction is simply a matter of holding the top of each rep and squeezing the calves for three to four counts before lowering the weight. This was very painful, but I always relished the muscle burn and felt it would only make me bigger. The pumping action would usually take place at the end of a set of, say, seated calf raises or leg press calf raises. After I couldn't do any more full-range-of-motion reps, I finished the set by doing short, quick reps (not quite all the way up or down) for as long as possible until my calves were screaming. I felt this action really chiseled the outer section of my calves for championship form."

Lou Ferrigno's Hulk Calves[2]

Being the Incredible Hulk wasn't the only thing incredible about Lou Ferrigno. His calves are pretty incredible as well. Use this routine to hulk out your own calves too.

Lou's Calf Routine:

Standing Calf Raise - Sets: 10-12, Reps: 6-10.
Seated Calf Raise - Sets: 10-12, Reps: 15-20.

Lou's advice on calf training in his own words:

. . .

"I like to devote one calf workout to the soleus muscle with seated calf raises (10 to 12 sets of 6 to 10 reps) and the next calf workout to the gastrocnemius with standing calf raises (10 to 12 sets of 15 to 20 reps)."

Tom Platz's Mega Calves[3]

Tom Platz is known for having some of the best legs of his generation, and any other. Although many remember his thighs, Tom's calves were the foundation upon which his phenomenal legs were built.

While Arnold is known for his preference for donkey calf raises, Tom preferred the static rep—holding a very heavy weight at full or partial extension—to help stimulate calf growth.

Tom's Calf Routine:

Standing Calf Raises - Sets: 3-4, Reps: 10-15.
Seated Calf Raises - Sets: 3-4, Reps: 10-15.
Hack Machine Calf Raises - Sets: 3-4, Reps: 10-15.
Static Calf Holds - Hold your maximum weight at full extension for as long as possible (e.g. seated on a leg press machine).

Tom's calf training in his own words:

"I'm going to tell you some stuff that I never really tell most people.

"Back in my day, everybody did calves like six days a week, but I had most success training calves twice a week. With my body type, really intense calf training twice a week proved to be most effective.

"I did normal calf raises, standing calf raises, seated calf raises primarily, those two major exercises. The one thing I did on the standing calf raise on certain days, and on the seated calf raise, at the end of my workout, I would put slowly and progressively, as many plates as possible. Joe Gold made a special seated calf machine, extended the bar so I could put ten 100-pound plates or fifteen 100-pound plates. My goal was to just hold the weight at the end of my workout. Many workouts I would just hold the weight, not up high, not real low, but in the middle. I would just hold it. Imagine just holding 1000 or 2000 pounds at the end of your routine, just holding it still until I could barely hold it.

"I'd have some of the monster guys in the gym push on it barely, watch me, stay close to me. As soon as I felt like it was getting too much and my tendons and ligaments couldn't handle the tension, I would say, "Take it now!" and they took it.

"My message to you is that the static rep, the partial static rep, maybe once a week, maybe twice a week at the most, proved to be unbelievable, magic for my calves. I never wanted to get implants. Between getting implants or doing heavy static partial work, the heavy training, hard work, old school training methodology worked best. That's the actual fact. I don't think I ever said that to a writer in a magazine. I may have. That works best for calves for me. One day I would do higher reps prior to that, of course, one day I did real low reps, and I alternated that. But, always, static reps proved to be most effective."

Erik Fankhouser's Mountainous Calves[4]

Erik has legendary calves. Unlike Arnold, Erik won the calf genetics lottery. But that hasn't stopped Erik from pushing his calves to their limits to achieve legendary gains.

Erik's Calf Routine:

. . .

Week 1:

Seated Calf Raise - Sets: 4, Reps: 12.
Leg Press Calf Raise - Sets: 4, Reps: 12.
Reverse Calf Raise - Sets: 4, Reps: 12.

Week 2:

One-leg Smith Machine Standing Calf Raise - Sets: 4, Reps: 15.
One-leg Donkey Calf Raise - Sets: 4, Reps: 15.
One-leg Reverse Calf Raise - Sets: 4, Reps: 15.

Erik's calf training in his own words:

"Yes, I've always had good calf development. I always tell people that I was 150 pounds and my calves were as big as they are now. They obviously weren't, but they were always pretty freaky. I had football-sized calves when I was in middle school. I've definitely brought them up through training, but at this point I'm not trying to add any more mass; just stimulate them to maintain what I have. They are my money-maker, so I have to keep them there."

James "Flex" Lewis's Superhero Calves[5]

Flex's calves are so impressive, he actually has to moderate his training to keep his body in balance. Here's an overview of one of Flex's calf training routines so you too can have monster calves.

Flex is an innovator who is constantly pushing himself with high-intensity training, coming up with new exercise variations and challenges, adapting to his needs while pushing his limits. His great calves are a result of these intensely dynamic efforts.

Lewis says, "My calf training is crazy."

After trying his workout, you'll see why.

Flex's Calf Routine:

Exercise	Sets	Reps
Leg press calf raises	4	25-35
Seated calf raises	4	25-35
Standing calf raises	3	25-35

Calf training tips from Flex:

• Before starting calf exercises, warm up and stretch your legs fully.

• Perform your reps quickly, the more the better. Weight is not the main consideration when training calves. The goal of the calf routine is to keep your blood flowing throughout the calf muscles while exercising.

• When training calves, find the optimal rhythm, timing, variations, and mix of movements to amplify your routine and development.

• Make sure your legs are fully pumped before stopping your calf routine. If your legs are too fatigued to do more reps with weight, use bodyweight calf raises to finish your calf workout.

Training calves with dedication has helped make the careers—and bodies—of the world's most elite bodybuilders. Even if you're not a bodybuilder, take the advice of some of the world's best bodybuilders to get your calves to grow!

CALF RAISES WITH STIFF-LEGGED JUMPS

Being intelligent about how you attack your calves is critical in capturing the muscle development you're after. Recognizing your calves are made up of different muscle groups and muscle fiber types, each which responds more readily to different stimuli, is critical to getting your calves to grow.

Use this dynamic superset to work your calves' slow and fast-twitch muscle fibers, hitting the muscles from different angles and speeds to shock them into growth:

1. **Standing Calf Raises** - Start this routine at the standing calf-raise machine. Do eight full, controlled reps. Make sure to pause for two-seconds at the bottom of each rep. Try to rest no longer than 10 to 15 seconds before moving on to the next movement. Having your barbell loaded and ready for your upcoming calf jumps will allow you to control rest times and keep your exercise tempo high.
2. **Weighted Calf Jumps** - Add roughly 25% of your body weight onto a barbell. Hold the loaded bar resting on your shoulders in a standing position as you would at the start of a squat and, with minimal knee bend and a neutral spine, jump up and down,

pushing up and through with the calves on each rep. Fully extend your toes downward as you jump upward to maximize your calves' engagement. Target 30 reps to start. The eccentric loading caused by the jumping and landing will encourage muscle growth.

3. **Repeat** - Perform the calf raise/calf jump superset combination four more times for five total sets.

As your strength improves, consider increasing the weight you use, the volume of your jumps, the height and intensity of your jumps, and the number of sets performed.

For variety, take your calf jumps outside using dumbbells or a weighted vest while performing single-leg calf raises on stairs or a curb. The ground, especially a grassed field, will be more forgiving on your joints.

The combination of calf raises and calf jumps should spur your calf growth to new heights.

STAIRWAY TO CALVES

The world is full of opportunities to build your calves. In writing *Killer Calves*, I hope to help you learn to see these opportunities too, and come up with many new growth-inducing variations that I haven't discovered. And —thankfully for your calves and the potential to help them grow—the world is also full of stairs.

Using stairs to help your calves grow is simple. Here's how you do it:

1. **Find suitable stairs**. If you don't have access to stairs, use a rock, a curb, or find a stable rectangular block… nothing should stop you from reaching your calf goals!
2. **Perform one-legged calf raises on the stairs using your bodyweight only.** Hold the stretch position for five seconds on every rep. Do five reps, then switch legs.
3. **Repeat.** Go up to the next step and perform single-leg calf raises for each leg.

Note: Try to find a set of stairs to do at least 50 reps per calf in a sequence, climbing up one step at a time after finishing each set with both legs. Going up one step at a time helps with your counting. That's 10 stairs at a minimum. There are no excuses... not even having no stairs!

Make this routine a habit and your calves will thank you for it.

If you have stairs in your house, do this twice a day.

If you don't have stairs, find an alternative.

Be warned, don't go crazy at first trying to build your calves using the stairs. Unless you've been working consistently with calf training, the soreness can be debilitating. You won't be able to walk or workout properly. And that will hurt your gains!

See the *Variations* chapter for more ways to push this program.

Consider anything from:

1. **Adding weights** - A weight vest works nicely to increase your workout's intensity while keeping the additional weight load aligned with your body structure throughout the movement.
2. **Increasing the number of stairs climbed** - More steps increases the number of sets performed.
3. **Increasing the number of reps performed on each step** - For example, doing 10 reps per leg instead of 5.
4. **Changing the timing or tempo of your reps** - Extending the stretch at the bottom of the rep and/or the contraction/hold at the top of the exertion. For example, a 5 or 10-second stretch or contraction held at full extension.
5. **Get creative!** - There are many other options to overcome your body's ability to adapt, from changing tempo, body orientation, and adding pauses mid-rep.

For example, one of my favorite variations is performing each rep with a 5 second contraction while wearing a weight vest. Maintaining the 50 total repetition target, do sets of 10 on each step finishing on the fifth step or keep pushing beyond 50 total reps. For additional fun—pain—hold your final contraction for as long as possible, such as a twenty count or whatever brings the burn. While doing this final contracted hold, lift up as high onto your toes as possible.

Remember, pushing yourself and your limits helps your calves grow!

MAXIMIZE TIME UNDER TENSION FOR CALF GAINS

Maximizing time under tension, the amount of time you are exerting during exercise, is a key ingredient to significant calf gains.

Calves can be a very challenging—and by challenging I mean frustrating—muscle group. If they don't have well-developed calves naturally, many people have to work their tails off to get them.

If you're reading this book, you're probably one of those hard gainers. To overcome the calf growth challenge, you need to combine quite a few factors to get the most effective stimulation.

Here are a few ways to build your calves by focusing on increased time under tension (the time spent working during sustained exertion without rest or recovery):

1. **Work your calves by combining heavy weights and high reps with very short rest periods between sets.** Perform calf circuits using different exercise angles to hit the muscles from various directions but be sure to keep the weights heavy and the reps high. For variations, add some tempo manipulation by moving

fast or slow through the exercise as well as adding pauses at your peak contraction and stretched position. Just because you've failed performing the full range of motion does not mean you cannot perform a portion of the exercise via a partial rep. Adding pulses at peak contraction after you can no longer push through the full exercise range will push your time under tension and help stimulate calf growth.

2. **Find a Smith machine and use it!** Perform Smith machine standing barbell calf raises. The stability-providing support posts from the Smith machine will let you lift heavy weights without losing movement quality from trying to balance the weight on your shoulders. Perform 12-15 reps per set to start. Hold a three-second pause at the peak calf contraction and a three-second pause at the stretch during the first or second half of your set for a simple exercise variation. Pause times can be changed based on weight used and your fitness level to maximize time under tension.

3. **Get creative with gym equipment.** Perform one-legged calf raises on the leg-press machine. Start with 12-15 reps per set. During the first half of the set, use a full range of motion using a complete stretch and toe extension as you push the weight. On the last half of the set, use partial extensions focusing on the top half of the movement. As with the Smith machine calf raises above, or when using other techniques from the *Variations* chapter, consider varying your exercise tempo to optimize your muscles' time under tension.

4. **Get off your feet, but don't rest!** Instead, go find a seated calf machine. Perform heavy seated calf raises to failure. Use variations discussed above including pulses, pauses and holds, adjusting the tempo of your lift, drop sets, and using various angles to hit the muscles from different sides.

5. **Sprint.** Sprinting is a great way to push your time under tension, especially as part of a larger calf program. After warming up, sprint 40 to 60 yards or meters, repeating your sprints 6 to 8 times. Sprint as fast as possible and then jog back to your starting point. Sprint twice per week and focus on running on

the balls of your feet as you go. Sprinting up hills makes the pain and growth even better. Vary your speed, distance, and rest times to add variety. See the chapter on sprinting and hill running for more ideas.

6. **Walk.** Yes, walk. Find the steepest hill you can. If you don't have a hill, use a treadmill set at the maximum incline setting, or simply use stairs. Walk briskly, as fast as possible, up the hill. Concentrate on engaging your calves as you walk and move through a complete range of motion with each step. Vary your tempo, going 20 to 30 seconds as fast as possible, then walk at a normal pace for the same amount of time. Add a backpack or weighted vest to push you during your hill or incline walks. Incorporate plyometric movements like skips and jumps for variation. Imagine you're hiking up a beautiful mountain to help those calves grow. The view from the top will be worth it!

To maximize your calf gains, you have to be willing to push them creatively. Whether that is through long, intense or frequent sets, while employing exercise variations in both, is up to you. As long as you give your body enough time to recover and avoid injury between sessions, maximizing time under tension is a surefire path to calf growth.

CALF RAISE AWAY TO BRING THE GAINS ALL DAY

Since calf muscles often respond well to exercises involving higher numbers of repetitions—due to their muscle fiber make-up and high physiologic stress tolerance—this high frequency training (HFT) program can help you improve your calf strength and enjoy more calf growth than you ever have before.

More than just an exercise routine to be done when you work out, think of this program as a slight lifestyle change, one in which you incorporate calf training daily. If you've already committed to exercising regularly, this routine is merely a calf-focused extension to that commitment.

High frequency single-leg calf raise program:

How Strong Are You? Before you begin this program, you need to determine your initial strength level. This evaluation requires an honest assessment of your initial strength. Since this is about you and you alone, do not cheat! You're performing this program for your betterment, not your ego. No one needs to know your results and you're not comparing yourself to anyone.

. . .

Calf Strength Test (Baseline strength):

To start, without shoes, perform one set of single-leg calf raises with each leg.

If at first the bare floor is too hard on your feet, carpet is fine, but you should work toward being comfortable on all surfaces.

Use as little assistance as possible to maintain your balance while performing your calf raises.

Use just your fingertips resting lightly on a countertop or against a wall to maintain your balance.

Try to perform 3 to 4 single-leg calf raises without holding onto anything to engage your ankle stabilizers to get a sense of the motion—the balance and stability required for the unassisted single-leg calf raises.

Take a short break and then see how many unassisted single-leg calf raises you can do with each leg. Go for it!

Tips:

1. Keep your exercising leg completely straight during every repetition to only engage your calf muscles. There should be no swaying or pumping via torso shifting or knee flexion to facilitate the calf raise.
2. Keep your body in a proper, vertical alignment while you lift.
3. Again, you are not trying to impress anyone, just to better yourself in the privacy of your own home or anywhere else you choose. This honest baseline assessment will show you how much opportunity you have to improve your functional strength and calf growth.
4. Note how many reps you perform with each leg. The goal here is at least 20 good clean reps, your baseline strength for each leg.

The Routine - This high-frequency training routine is the heart of the program, the one that will boost your strength and your calves with it.

Perform 3 sets of single-leg calf raises with as many reps as possible (AMRAP) with each leg every day, at morning, midday, and night using the techniques outlined in the initial strength test, such as straight legs, no skipping/cheating, and minimal support. Push yourself to see those results! Technique tips:

Begin with your stronger calf to help create your target goals, as you want each calf as strong as the other, establishing neural carryover to your weaker side, making you stronger and more goal focused.

Perform each calf raise slowly. Drive up through the ball of your foot onto your big toe and reach the highest elevation possible by squeezing your calf muscle to peak tension. Hold the raise at full extension for 2 seconds with each rep.

Maintain good posture via a long, relaxed spine, to help facilitate proper form and reduce risks of cramping while exercising.

Spread the sets evenly throughout the day. Perform one set in the morning, one in the afternoon, and one in the evening. There is no break for great calves!

Do not perform any additional calf training in your normal workouts.

Perform the sets barefoot to maximally engage your calves through a complete range of motion. You can wear shoes of course. Just make sure to get all your sets in, whether at work, home, or wherever possible.

Stop your set once your knee flexes, you can no longer stabilize, or your ability to elevate onto your toes decreases by one inch (two centimeters).

Rest for 30 seconds between each side.

Do this routine every day for two weeks.

The Retest - You've committed to your calves for two weeks. Now you get to see how far you've come!

After 2 weeks of daily calf training, the time has come to retest your standing, single-leg calf raise performance.

Before testing, take one full day off from calf raises.

The following day, after 48 hours from your last set of calf raises, retest your standing single-leg calf raise following the guidelines above—good form, maintain body alignment, and no cheating—with **one** exception. Do not include the 2-second peak contraction in the test sets. Otherwise, perform a normal set of as many reps as possible.

If you still fall short of the 20-repetition target, continue with the daily program for two more weeks and retest again.

Depending on your performance, keep extending the program until you reach your goal, if you achieve the goal with one leg but not the other.

Keep Pushing! - You are not done! There are many more goals and variations ahead if you decide to keep pushing and improving in your single-leg calf training.

New targets:

You could work toward performing standing single-leg calf raises *without any* balance assistance.

You could work toward performing unassisted single-leg calf raises with your opposite knee raised up, your opposite leg forward, backward, or out to the side.

You could incorporate this program into your exercise routine indefinitely to keep pushing those gains.

Use variations to increase your limits, increase your strength, and boost your growth further.

While exercises with strict form are a great place to start your single-leg program, variations can help push your improvements over the top. Options include:

1. Pulsing at the top of your contraction motion after reaching the point where you can no longer perform full reps, to maximize the burn and muscle fatigue.
2. Destabilizing your body by leaning slightly forward or backward to force your muscles to fire and contract in new ways as you perform reps.
3. Slowing down the contraction (lifting) and relaxation (lowering) sections of your calf raises.
4. Holding the peak contraction for longer than 2 seconds.
5. Adding weight while maintaining strict form.

6. Never letting your heel touch the ground to maintain tension throughout each set.
7. Incorporating any other suggestions mentioned in the *Variations* chapter.

If you question that a seemingly simple program like this one works, just look at the calf development of almost any ballet dancer. You'll see real-world proof that unassisted calf raises on the floor, lifting consistently at high volume, will do wonders for your calf development.

Once you're able to perform 10 perfect, single-leg calf raises unassisted while holding a 2-second peak contraction at the top of each rep, you will achieve an above average level of calf size and strength. From there, using the continued supplemental options outlined above, you can leave *normal* far behind.

THE DANCER'S CALF-TRAINING ANSWER

If you look across all athletic groups as a whole and evaluate them by calf aesthetics—particularly relative to body size and shape—to determine which group has the best calves, you would be hard-pressed to find a group with better calves than dancers.

Good cases for the best athletes' calves could also be made for sprinters —track and field and cycling—and gymnasts.

Dancers, too, have amazing calves. When you compare dancers' calves against those of many gym-goers, you will agree that the dancers' greatest strength is many gym-goers' most glaring weakness.

So, if you've tried almost every calf-training approach known to both man and gym monsters—drop sets, reverse drop sets, plyometrics, negative-accentuated/eccentric training, explosive movements/concentric training, extended sets, isometrics, tempo adjustments, extended burns, supersets, tri-sets and giant sets, escalating density training, partial reps, training with perfect form, unilateral training, stair climbing, hill sprints, high-intensity interval training, farmer's carries, and any other program or idea the gym gods can summon—you may want to consider training your calves like a dancer.

You can still train the rest of your body like the Incredible Hulk but take your calf cues from the amazing legs of dancers. Then your whole body will hulk out.

Dancer's Calves

Dancers are constantly using their calves, consistently and repetitively up on their toes, holding their calves contracted at full extension while balancing on the balls of their feet. They are jumping explosively over and over while focusing the effort into their calves. and moving up and down with precision as well as explosion. Dancers, as much as any athlete, are performing more bodyweight calf raises than just about anyone else.

In ballet, lifting up onto your toes using bodyweight calf raises is known as relevé. For you, lifting up onto your toes is called calf gains.

I'm are not asking you to wear a tutu—though you can if you so wish—but I am asking you to consider calf training like someone who wears a tutu. If you want to experience the calf hypertrophy effects of a dancer, and enjoy their excellent calf development, then start your dancer training today.

The solution is simple: perform at least 100 reps of daily bodyweight calf raises. As with the three-times-a-day single-leg calf-training program from the last chapter, the dancer's calf program can be considered a life-style choice incorporated into your daily routines.

Do this dancer's calf program every day and watch your spindly chop-sticks transform into tree trunks.

The Dancer's Calf Program:

Standing calf raises on the floor:

Begin your dancer's calf program by performing 50 repetitions of calf raises from the floor.

The goal is to work up to at least 100 reps using only your bodyweight.

Perform this workout religiously every day for a month. Not only will your calves grow but also, your balance and coordination will improve.

Proper form when performing your standing calf raises is very important.

Stand with your feet roughly shoulder-width apart, angling your toes slightly outward. Concentrate on raising your heels straight upward without flexing your knees or bouncing your body up and down as you lift. As you exert, try to isolate as much tension into your calves as possible. This is how your calves grow!

Contract your calves hard at the top of each exertion. Try not to hold onto anything for support. This will only limit your load and your gains with it. Avoiding assistance will also make sure your stabilizing muscles are fully engaged and become stronger. To limit assistance and involve stabilizing muscles, let your arms relax by your sides or place your hands on your hips. If you need to hold your arms up or out to assist with balance, that is fine.

Perform the exercises in bare feet without shoes. This will allow a greater range of motion and force you to involve more muscles as you work. Raise your heels as high as possible off the ground. Be sure to distribute your weight evenly over the entirety of the balls of your feet and toes. Hold the top contraction at full extension for at least 2 seconds. Do not cheat or bounce! You must pause, coming to a defined stop at the peak contraction. You *must* feel a contraction in the calves as you hold at the top of the exercise.

Lower slowly in a controlled fashion. Don't just plop back to the ground as though you're falling onto the couch after work. If you don't raise and lower correctly, the rep doesn't count. These calf raises have to be quality repetitions to get the most from this type of training—quality reps with quality form = gains. Not only will your primary gastrocnemius calf muscles burn, but so will your stabilizing muscles as well. Hitting all these muscles will make huge differences to your calf development.

This program will take about 10 minutes a day over a month to start seeing results. Each controlled repetition will take about 6 seconds in total, 2 seconds to raise, 2 seconds held at the peak contraction, and 2 seconds to lower with no pause at the bottom. Since you'll be performing roughly 100 reps per day, you'll be working your calves for about 10 minutes daily. Throw in stretching and any cooldown and you'll add another minute or more. A small sacrifice with proven results.

Aside from getting massive calves, this program has the benefit of being doable anywhere at any time. No special equipment or memberships are required. All that is needed is your commitment and effort to see great gains.

Keep working and challenging yourself until you reach a level of calf development you're satisfied with relative to your goals. Then consider reducing your workload to 2 to 3 sessions a week to maintain those gains or keep pushing for more. If you return to using other equipment for your calves, just one session a week should help maintain your new development and give you a break from potential boredom. For other bonus options to keep those challenges and gains coming, see below.

Bonus Work for Bonus Gains:

Once you have completed your first full month of the dancer calf program, add an additional 5, 10, or 20 pounds using a weighted vest, dumbbell, kettlebell, or plate, and go at it again. If the standing calf raises are too easy for you at any time, think about adding additional weight earlier in the program.

Use other variations in addition to, or as an alternative to, more weight. For example, add a longer peak contraction at the top of your raise, slow the rate you lift and lower your body, lift your arms overhead to change the balance component, or increase the number of repetitions performed.

Be prepared to work through the burn. Once you come out of the fire on the other side, your calves will thank you.

And even dancers will be envious.

HIT THE HILLS FOR GREAT CALVES (AND LEGS)

The hills are alive with calves!

If you want to build calf muscles quickly, hill sprints are a great way to go.

To start, find a hill that is about 50 to 200 yards or meters long. If you live in an area that is relatively flat and doesn't have any suitable hills, use a treadmill set on a steep incline over the same distance for similar results. Stairs are also an option as long as there are enough flights to challenge you.

Take time to warm up sufficiently before starting your hill routine—your hamstrings, muscles, and tendons will all benefit. Whether that's walking and jogging up the hill or around the area, dynamic stretching, jumping jacks, or running in place, be prepared for the amount of difficult exertion required by hill running.

Hill Running Overview:

Now that you've found a suitable hill and have warmed up, sprint up the hill close to your maximum speed and strength. When running, be sure you're moving through full extension with your feet to fully activate the calves. Run in a natural upright posture, keeping your neck, back, and shoulders relaxed, trying not to lean forward into the hill. When you reach the top of the hill, let your momentum continue for a few yards or meters, relaxing and letting the tension out of your muscles as you slow down.

Then, jog back down the hill.

Repeat the drill 5 to 10 times, or more if you're ready and want to push yourself.

As you become more comfortable with hill running, bump up the intensity and volume and add in more variations.

Complete Basic Sprint Workout with Warmup:

Directions: With dynamic stretching—active movements where your joints and muscles go through a full range of motion to prepare for exertion—perform each moving 'stretch' for at least two seconds (e.g. legs swings, hip circles, arm circles, torso twists, walking knee to chest raises, straight leg kicks, etc. should each last a couple of seconds as you move dynamically through the stretch), and repeat each dynamic movement to get your body ready. When sprinting, your rests and recovery periods are between each sprint, and determined by how long you take to jog or walk back down the hill. But remember, don't draw your breaks out too much.

Warmup:

1. **Walking hamstring stretch** - Perform the dynamic stretch while walking for 10 yards or meters. Bend at the waist, holding your forward leg straight and reach your hands toward the ground by your forward foot with each step. Keep the non-stretching knee bent slightly for stability as you stretch.
2. **Walking groiner stretch** - Perform this dynamic stretch while striding forward for 10 yards or meters. For each lunging stride,

take a big step as if you're performing a lunge and drop your back knee toward the ground. As you settle into the stretch, keep your head up as you bring your chest toward your extended knee. Place both hands on the ground so you don't lose balance as you stretch. Lean forward as needed to bring the stretch deeper into your hamstrings and glutes.

3. **Walking quad stretch** - Perform the stretch while walking forward for 10 meters or yards. While standing, take one foot and pull it upward toward your buttocks. Alternating legs, drop your foot, take one step forward, and then repeat the quad stretch.

4. **Low hurdle running drill** - Perform the exercise for 25 meters or yards. Run forward and imagine you're running over a low, 4 to 6-inch (10 to 15 centimeter) high hurdle with each step.

5. **High hurdle running drill** - Perform the warmup exercise for 25 meters or yards. Run forward and visualize striding over a 12-inch (1/3 meter) high hurdle with each step.

6. **Leg swings** - Perform 10 swings per leg, swinging your legs front to back and side to side. When swinging your legs, stand upright, keep your leg straight, and hold onto something stable. Swing each leg 10 times backward and forward and then 10 times side to side while maintaining good form. Switch legs when complete.

The Workout:

1. **Uphill sprint** - Run uphill for 10 seconds, roughly 25 to 50 meters or yards, this will help reduce lactic acid buildup in your legs. Use 80 to 100 percent of your maximum effort when sprinting.

2. **Repeat** - Perform the hill sprint 6 times using good form while fully engaging your muscles, especially your calves.

Ramping Intensity Sprint Program:

Implementing many variations for your hill workouts will build your calves. Here's a graduated routine that builds in intensity going farther and higher over time, while reducing set volume for longer distances:

1. 5 sprints x 10 meters or yards, rest for 15 seconds between sprints.
2. 4 sprints x 20 meters or yards, rest for 30 seconds between sprints.
3. 3 sprints x 30 meters or yards, rest for 60 seconds between sprints.
4. 2 sprints x 40 meters or yards, rest for 90 seconds between sprints.
5. 1 sprint x 50 plus meters or yards. Go farther if the hill is long enough and you're ready to challenge yourself.

Remember, the emphasis when sprinting is on exercise quality despite the high exertion. To give adequate recovery time, the rest periods between sets increases with each new distance. The better your form and the more engaged you are in your movements, the better your results... be intense but maintain good form!

Reduce your volume and intensity if you are inexperienced with sprinting. As you get fitter, increase the distances, variation, and intensity—or decrease the rest intervals—to help prevent plateauing. For example, run longer, harder, use a steeper hill, or add weight to continue overloading your muscles. In addition to more developed calves, be prepared for some serious back, leg, and core development as well as a leaner overall physique.

The Never-Ending Sets Workout:

. . .

This hill program relies on increasing the number, intensity, and length of sprints as your strength and endurance increases.

As you adjust to this method of high-volume sprint training, the running intervals become longer, increasing in duration to 10 to 12 seconds per sprint. When beginning, look for a hill about 40 meters or yards long. Find a bigger hill as needed.

Warmup:

To warm up for your sprints, do cardio, light jogging, and dynamic stretches for roughly 10 to 15 minutes. Short jogs, leg swings, jumping jacks, skips, and squats are good examples of exercises to help you get ready.

The workout:

1. When you feel ready, perform five uphill sprints at roughly 70 to 80 percent of maximal effort over roughly 40 meters or yards.
2. Shake out your legs to remain loose and let yourself recover as you walk down the hill after each sprint.
3. Finish your workout with a 10-to-15 minute cool down using exercises and stretches similar to those used for the warmup.
4. As you train and improve, gradually increase your sprints' length, intensity, and number by one or two sprints per week until you've progressed to 20 at maximal effort over a longer distance. Each sprint should take about 10 seconds to complete.

The Mountain:

. . .

This program is as simple as it is grueling. Find a hill, the bigger and steeper the better, but one that you can run up. Bring something heavy, such as a weight vest, a sandbag, a loaded backpack, a bag of dog food, last year's tax forms, or whatever works. Warm up thoroughly. Once you're ready, holding your weight securely, run up the hill as fast as you can. When you can't run, walk. When you can't walk, scramble and crawl.

If you don't have a long, steep hill nearby, use a treadmill set on maximum gradient.

If you don't have a treadmill, use stairs. You will need enough flights to push yourself to your limits.

The goal of the mountain is to reach absolute failure in a single set. Use good form and push through with your calves with each step—as long as you're able—while your muscles and form slowly deteriorate.

The Mountain is not a workout to be undertaken lightly. It is intended to push and test your limits... two key factors in both physical and mental growth.

Hill Sprint Tips & Tricks:

1. If your hill is close to your home, consider walking, jogging, or bicycling to the hill as a warm-up. Then walk, jog, or cycle back home as a cool-down.
2. If you find your sprinting area has poor traction, consider a pair of track shoes or cleats to improve your grip. Alternatively, if your hill is part of a trail, you may want to purchase trail running shoes to maintain good footing and provide ankle support.
3. Use whatever hill(s) you have nearby to set your target sprint distances. If you have two or more hills close, create separate workouts for each hill. Alternatively, adjust the length of your sprint workouts each week based on the hills available—long and short hill-sprinting sessions.

4. Time your sprints with a stopwatch. To help prevent injury, when your times decrease by 10 percent or more, stop your session for the day.

5. Because of their intensity, allow yourself adequate time to recover between hill workouts.

6. As your strength and stamina increase, add more sprints per session.

7. Try other sprint programs to add variety, intensity, and prevent plateauing.

8. To make your sessions more intense, add weight. Weight vests are a nice option, particularly those that offer adjustable weight ranges. Start low and work up to higher weights.

9. Hills also offer great opportunities for other exercises, so consider adding them to your routine since you've already come this far. Options include hill jumps—jumping up the hill for quads and glutes—decline crunches, bear crawls up and down the hill, and incline/decline push-ups. Now that you've found your hill, make the most of it!

10. Use variations in how you sprint. Run pushing up from the ground using a full range of motion in your feet to emphasize calf engagement. As an alternative, stay on your toes as you run. Mix techniques to keep your muscles firing and prevent your calves from adapting.

11. If you don't have access to hills, stairs, a treadmill, or if you just want some variety in your program, consider doing any of these hill sprint workouts on flat ground.

Hill sprinting is a powerful tool to bring to your calf-training arsenal. Not only will you get outside for a change of scenery and pace, but also, your calves will never know what hit them.

SIFF LUNGES AND SIFF SQUATS FOR DIAMOND CALVES

If you're frustrated about not getting your desired results in your calves even though you work your legs diligently, have I got an exercise variation for you!

Siff lunges and Siff squats!

Here's a program that will put your calves under pressure, polish them, and eventually turn them into diamonds:

Siff lunges - Siff lunges are a unique lunge variation where you always stay on the tips of your toes. To perform a Siff lunge, elevate off your heels and remain on your toes throughout the exercise. Siff lunges can also be performed plyometrically as well for an intensified variation—jumping up and down through your lunges while remaining on your toes throughout the movement. For your Siff lunge routine, perform:

1. **Sets**: 3-4.
2. **Reps**: 8-10 per side.
3. **Rest**: 90 seconds between sets.

Standing calf raises - Perform your standing calf raises on a calf-raise machine, using a squat bar, on a seated leg press machine, or with dumb-bells... whatever makes you work. For your standing calf raises, perform:

1. 2 sets of 6 to 8 reps with your feet in the neutral, forward-facing position.
2. 2 sets of 6 to 8 reps with your feet and toes turned outward.
3. 2 sets of 6 to 8 reps with your feet and toes turned inward.

Be sure to start each repetition from a pause in the stretched position. For added burn, pause at the peak contraction as well.

Seated calf raises - Perform your seated calf raises on a seated calf raise machine. If you don't have access to a seated calf machine, use a chair, elevating your heels off the ground using a plate, bar, or other flat object and rest the weights on your knees to lift. Alternatively, squat down with your knees completely bent and your buttocks resting on your heels, and perform calf raises from the seated squat position. For your seated calf raises, perform:

1. **Sets**: 3.
2. **Reps**: Perform 30 total repetitions. Do 10 reps with your feet and toes turned inward, 10 reps with your feet and toes in a neutral, forward-facing position, and 10 reps with your feet and toes turned outward.

Notes:

1. Each set of seated calf raises has a total of 30 repetitions.
2. For the seated and standing calf raises, start each rep from a

stretched position at the bottom of the lift and hold the peak top contraction for at least two seconds.

Perform this calf-burning routine two to three times per week.

If your calves have lost their luster, this routine will put some shine on those gems.

Bonus Siff Exercise:

For an added bonus, throw in Siff squats on your leg day(s) to get your calves screaming.

How to Siff Squat:

Start your leg workouts with Siff squats. Siff squats are performed exactly like regular squats with two exceptions: you stay on the balls of your feet while squatting and you use a slightly lighter weight than in a normal squat.

To do your Siff squats, use 75 to 85 percent of the weight you would typically use for a standard squat. Start your set as you would for a normal squat with the bar resting on your shoulders. After getting into the start position, raise your heels off the ground so that you're standing on the balls of your feet. Use a block or bar if needed as a guide to help keep your heels off the ground or for stability. Perform a squat, keeping your heels elevated for the entire movement.

Perform 2 to 3 sets of 8 to 10 reps each. Rest for two minutes between sets. Stay on your toes as much as possible to engage your calves and stability muscles.

. . .

Why the Siff Squat Works:

The classic squat is one of the best overall total body-building exercises because it engages numerous muscle groups for maximum stimulus and hormone release. In addition to all the benefits of traditional squats, Siff squats force your calves to support a heavier load than normal, providing a powerful stimulus for growth. Siff squats also add additional stress and growth opportunities for your quads because raising your heels forces your center of gravity and weight slightly forward during exertion.

The dynamic Siff squat can help strengthen your weak points and push your body to its limits.

JUMP FOR JOY FOR YOUR CALVES

Jumping explosively can be great for your calves and body in general. Plyometrics—jumping exercises—are an excellent tool to increase strength, explosive power, and muscle mass. Here are a few calf-focused plyometric exercises to push your calves in new directions and help them grow.

These exercises can be worked into your calf routine, incorporated into your leg days, or used together to build a routine of their own. Alternatively, add them with other plyometric exercises to boost your overall leg strength and power.

Be careful when performing jumping exercises as they put quite a lot of pressure and stress on your joints and body. As with sprints, warm up thoroughly before beginning plyometric training. Listen to your body and take precautions to reduce injury risk. Taking precautions such as jumping on a mat or grass and using good form can all reduce impact pressures.

Ankle Jumps:

Ankle jumps are a classic calf workout that is both explosive and athletic. When doing ankle jumps, take inspiration from sprinters, dancers, and gymnasts. Ankle jumps mimic these athletes' explosive activity, taking your calves to new heights.

Here's how:

1. Stand with your feet together with your arms relaxed and your hands resting loosely by your sides.
2. Keeping your legs as straight as possible, jump up and down from a single spot by pushing explosively off your toes. Jump as high as possible with maximum effort and exertion. Do not let your heels touch down onto the ground between jumps.
3. Continue jumping until your calves burn and your form starts to become compromised.
4. Rest and repeat until failure.

Tips and Variations:

1. Jump from side to side to work the lateral sides of your calves.
2. To increase the intensity of the workout, incorporate any of the methods listed. Increasing the number of reps or sets, try hopping on one leg, wearing a weighted vest, jumping higher, or holding dumbbells while carrying out your jumps.
3. Remember, ankle jumps are not a squat jump or normal leap. Avoid bending at the knees as much as possible when performing your ankle jumps to keep the focus of your exertion in your calf muscles as much as possible.

Jumping Rope:

. . .

If you want to take your calves to new heights, jump into plyometrics for a world of exercises to push yourself to new limits. Jumping rope is a plyometric classic where you can isolate your calves to your heart's content. Although typically associated with adding definition to your calves and legs in general, jumping rope can also build your calves depending on your program and goals. When jumping, use a full range of motion and focus primarily on your calves to get better muscle engagement and improved results.

Basic Jump Rope Routine:

To start your jump rope workouts, consider alternating between 30 seconds of work with 30 seconds of rest. Taken together, each exercise and rest cycle makes one round. Do 10 to 20 rounds in total, choosing from the jump rope variations outlined below.

As you progress, perform each exercise for a minute or more with shorter rests in between. Build up your exertion phases as your skill, endurance, and strength grow. Harder exercises like double-unders may be more difficult to sustain for the designated time. Just do your best and keep working.

Jump Rope Variations:

1. **Basic Jump** - The classic jump rope option. Simply jump up and down in place as you swing the rope around and under your feet. The basic jump is easy to perform and doing it for longer intervals will get a good calf burn. Adjust the height and speed of your jumps to increase intensity.
2. **Front-to-Back** - Jump forward and backward as you jump over the rope. With this jump, your body has to dynamically stabilize as you're moving your feet forwards and backwards. This

movement gives your calves an extra challenge, targeting more muscle fibers.

3. **Side-to-Side** - Jump from side to side laterally while jumping over the rope. Side jumps improve your lateral speed and explosiveness. These explosive movements can improve muscle definition and density.

4. **Alternating Foot Steps** - Alternate between landing on each foot as you jump from one leg to the other while jumping over the rope. This variation is performed as if you are running in place. The quick tempo helps improve your calves' reaction time.

5. **High Knee Step** - Perform alternating jumps over the rope as you would with alternating foot step jumps, except with this variation, raise your feet and knees higher, aiming for knees bent with thighs parallel to the ground. This is a higher impact exercise, so it improves calf strength.

6. **Single-Leg Jumps** - Jump up and down on one leg without alternating between feet. Single-leg jumps are great for explosiveness and strength because you're putting all of your bodyweight and impact energy on one leg, isolating each calf. All the energy involved in jumping on one leg will also work your feet and ankles.

7. **Double-Unders** - Jump into the air high enough to swing the jump rope beneath your feet twice before landing. The higher jumps from double-unders will improve power and explosiveness.

8. **Mummy Kicks** - Alternate kicking your feet out forward as you jump and stay on the balls of your feet and toes the whole time. With mummy kicks, your feet kick outward with legs mostly straight and then return to their starting position below the body in preparation to jump outward again. This exercise is calf muscle intensive. Focus on contracting your calves every time your feet hit the ground.

As with any jumping exercise, consider adding weight, such as with a weighted vest or increasing your jumping height to increase intensity. If needed, try jumping on a mat or other soft surface to reduce the stress of impact on your joints.

Jump Rope Circuit Routine:

There's a wealth of options to choose from to create a calf-burning jump rope workout. Here's a great circuit incorporating the jump rope variations.

Do the following exercises in a complete circuit 2 or 3 times. Rest for 10 seconds in between each jump rope exercise in the circuit before moving on to the next movement.

1. 30-second basic jump – a standard two-footed jump.
2. 30-second alternating footsteps – jump as though you're running in place.
3. 60-second single-leg jumps – 30-second jump on one leg before switching to the other leg for a further 30 seconds.
4. 30-second mummy kicks – kicking feet forward as you jump.
5. 30-second double-unders – rotate the rope twice with each jump.
6. 30-second single leg double-unders – 30 seconds with each leg. If you can't do single leg double-unders, repeat the double leg double-unders or do more single leg jumps.

Add variations to keep challenging yourself and to increase the intensity. Again, adding a weight vest and higher jumps will also push your calves harder.

Explosive, Nonjumping Calf Exercise Routine:

. . .

You don't have to jump off the ground to mimic the explosive exertions of leaping into the air. This routine mimics the forceful movements and dynamic pressures associated with leaping and sprinting to blast your calves into the strata.

Be sure to keep your knees straight but not locked out during each of these exercises.

Single-Leg Explosive Calf Raises:

1. Stand on a block, stair, or platform with the heel of one foot hanging over the edge.
2. Slowly lower your heel while keeping your knee straight.
3. Explosively extend your ankle upward as far as your range of motion allows, pushing upward through the ball of your foot and onto your toes as you lift.
4. Be sure to pause at the bottom of the exercise to reduce Achilles tendon involvement and encourage full muscle engagement.
5. Perform 3 sets for each leg with 6 to 8 explosive reps per set.

Single-Leg Hurdle Jumps:

1. Place 6 to 8 agility or speed-training hurdles in a straight line along the ground. Set each hurdle roughly 2 feet (2/3 of a meter) apart. If you don't have hurdles, visualize jumping over a low object—about one to three inches / two to eight centimeters above the ground—as you bounce forward. Alternatively, place other small objects on the ground to jump over.
2. On one leg, jump over the hurdles one at a time without pausing between jumps, traveling over the hurdles as quickly as possible.

3. Perform 2 to 3 sets with 6 to 8 repetitions for each leg. Do all the jumps in a set with the same leg before switching to the other leg.

Single-Leg Box Jumps:

1. Stand on one leg with a 4 to 6-inch (10 to 15 centimeter) box, block, or step in front of you.
2. Jump up onto the box, powerfully forcing your foot downward to generate power and upward momentum.
3. Jump down and quickly explode upward again to repeat.
4. Perform 3 sets with 6 to 8 repetitions for each leg.

For each of these exercises, consider adding height or weight for additional intensity.

These are but a few of the many jumping exercises that will blast your calves. For more ideas, take inspiration from your childhood when you jumped and skipped for fun. Also, look to track athletes' plyometric training, particularly those of sprinters, long-jumpers, and high-jumpers for additional ideas. Basketball drills, particularly those with a plyometric emphasis, are another great source of ideas for plyometric training.

Now go out and get jumping for those calf gains!

BLOOD FLOW RESTRICTION TO RELEASE CALF GROWTH

This book is full of exercises and ideas to help you get a skin-splitting amount of blood flowing to your calves. Choices to torture your legs and get those calves to grow include high volume training, explosive training, heavy training, drop sets, reverse drop sets, supersets, partial sets, plyometrics, and numerous others.

But one of the most effective ways to influence your muscles' pump is through blood flow restriction (BFR) or occlusion training.

Knee wraps offer a simple, easily accessible means to use BFR training on the calves. Simply apply the wraps just below the knee, right above where the gastrocnemius muscle meets the knee joint. Tighten the wraps about 30 to 40 percent looser than you would for a set of squats. Experiment with the tension until the tightness feels most comfortable to you, especially if you have never used wraps before.

Wrapping makes each set more challenging. If you wrap your calves too tightly, you'll never complete a full set—you have been warned!

Use any exercise or machine to train with your legs wrapped, including seated calf raises, donkey calf raises, horizontal calf extensions, or standing calf raises.

If you're truly working, be prepared to test your physical and mental limits when you exercise your calves using BFR.

When working your calves with BFR, aim for three sets of 10 to 15 repetitions with 30-second rest breaks in between each set. The intensity of the burn you'll get with BFR calf training will challenge your resolve. To help with recovery and calf development, be sure to stretch in between sets and after—massage, heat, cold packs, and electrical muscle stimulation are other valuable recovery options.

Here's a basic overview of how BFR training works:

1. Do 10 to 15 full range reps.
2. Stand and rest/stretch for 30 seconds.
3. Perform another set of 10 to 15 reps.
4. Rest/stretch another 30 seconds.
5. Finish with a final set of 10 to 15 reps.
6. Then remove the wraps.

Work up to three rounds of these calf killers.

When undertaking BFR training, don't forget the second key to calf hypertrophy—stretching. A good 30-second stretch of each calf at the end of each set of BFR is both painful and vital.

Since you're performing standard calf raises with your legs wrapped, consider any variation presented in this book to increase the intensity of your exercise or shift the emphasis as you train with BFR—rep timing and cadence, contractions, pauses, weight amount, number of reps, rep explosivity or wrap tightness. If lifting heavier weights, consider dropping the number of reps as well.

Your calves will thank me when you're done… once the pain subsides.

MORE CALF ROUTINES AND TECHNIQUES

I hope *Killer Calves* has your brain bursting with ideas of ways to boost and enhance your calf development. I also hope this book has inspired you to become just as stubborn as your calves and willing to do everything you possibly can to get them to grow without giving up.

Additionally, I hope that the programs and variations in *Killer Calves* have given you enough information to begin exploring new calf-blasting routines of your own.

However, in case you need more, here are a few bonus calf-destroying programs to keep you pushing, and calf raising to your ultimate goals—killer calves.

The Two-Minute Calf Raise

This standing calf-raise routine aims to maximize your benefits from using the standing calf-raise machine, helping you overcome bad habits or poor form you may have developed in the past.

This routine requires you to leave your ego at the door. As you get stronger, you'll eventually be able to add more weight and find other ways to intensify the routine.

Here's how:

1. Choose a weight 50 to 75% lighter than you would generally use for a set of 10 to 15 reps.
2. Do your first rep with a nice hard contraction at the highest point of your lift, and then lower your heels until you're in a complete stretch at the bottom of the lift. <u>Important</u>: You are constantly controlling the weight on the way down and not dropping it. Actively resist the weight pushing down into the calves as you lower, feeling the weight in your calves as you move. Hold the stretched bottom position for at least 10 seconds. Use a clock if you have to but don't cut your time short!
3. Now do another long, controlled rep. That means raise up, squeeze tightly, control the weight down to full extension, and hold at the bottom for another full 10-second stretch.
4. Perform 12 to 15 of these slow, controlled repetitions. If you performed the reps properly, your calves will have been under two minutes or more of unrelenting tension.
5. Perform 3 total sets of slow, extended calf raises.
6. Wonder when you'll be able to walk again. Just kidding… walking and stretching will help relieve the soreness and stiffness. And the pain will remind you why you're putting yourself through this torture.
7. For variations, consider holding the contractions at the top of your raise longer, adding additional weight, or increasing the number of reps performed.

Sprinting Intervals

· · ·

As an alternative to hill sprints, consider doing sprinting intervals on flat ground.

Why, you might ask?

The powerful legs of sprinters can rival those of some bodybuilders. Sprinting is an anaerobic exercise, meaning sprints do not rely on oxygen consumption during exertion and mainly utilize fast-twitch muscle fibers. Sprinting creates an ideal framework for calf growth since sprinting requires rapid deceleration which results in powerful eccentric muscle contractions. It also harnesses significant power with each explosive movement and utilizes rapid acceleration, creating forceful concentric contractions as your legs propel your body. In addition to calf growth, sprinting will also give you further muscular development in your quads, hamstrings, glutes, and core, as well as improving your cardiovascular resilience.

How to Sprint:

The biomechanics of sprinting are a bit different than regular running or jogging. With traditional jogging, you are striking the ground heel to toe with each stride. In contrast, sprinting will have you striking the ground with your toes first. This toe-first strike is where the eccentric contraction of the calf muscles comes in. Depending on your speed and form, you may or may not even touch your heels to the ground during sprints.

When sprinting, focus on landing on your toes instead of your heels. Perform a series of intervals with a moderate to high work-to-rest ratio—short exertions and longer rests. For example, you might sprint for 10 to 20 seconds at maximum speed and rest for 2 to 3 minutes between each sprint.

For variations, perform any of the hill sprint routines—mentioned previously—on flat ground, add weight, increase sprint distance, incorporate plyometrics, or reduce the rest time between sets.

Seated Calf Scorchers

. . .

If you like to work your calves at the end of your workout but your legs are so burned out that you can barely stand, then this timed seated calf raise workout is for you.

Here's how:

1. On the seated calf machine, perform as many repetitions as you can in a full minute. You are not counting reps. You are pushing yourself hard for a full minute.
2. Use good form and a controlled eccentric—negative downward movement.
3. Do not stop exercising for the entire minute.
4. Do at least 2 sets, focusing on getting the maximum amount of work in each minute.
5. Get a fire extinguisher ready to put out your calves. Or stretch. I recommend stretching.
6. Add more weight, change the angles of your feet, or increase the exercise duration, which will increase the number of reps performed, to intensify the set.

2-day Trauma

If you want your calves to grow, to be strong, and give your body foundational stability, then this 2-day program is just what you need.

You'll perform this calf routine twice a week, and also take a 48-hour break between the High and Low Volume sections. Session 1 focuses on low weight with high volume. Session 2 focuses on heavy weight with low volume. Both routines will light your calves on fire. And, combined, they will help your calves grow.

. . .

Here's how:

Day 1 - High-Volume

The high-volume day consists of two separate supersets.

Perform the seated calf raises and donkey calf raises detailed below in succession with a 10-second rest between each exercise to make the first high-volume superset. Rest for 2 minutes between supersets. Repeat the seated calf raises and donkey calf raises in sequence for a total of 3 super-sets using the appropriate number of reps for that set.

Move to the standing calf raise for 10 sets using a 10-second break between sets as explained below.

Seated Calf Raises - Perform 3 sets x 10-5-5 reps, respectively. This means you'll do 10 reps in the first set, then 5 reps in both the second and third sets. Use a 1-0-1 rhythm for your lifts. That means you will take 1 second to lower the weight down. You will not pause at the bottom of the lift. And you will take 1 second to raise the weight back up.

Donkey Calf Raises - Do 3 sets x 30-50 reps in each set. Perform each lift with a 1-0-1 rhythm, as explained above.

Standing Calf Raises - Perform 10 sets x 10-30 reps each set. Use a 1-1-1 tempo for each lift. This means you will take 1 second to lower the weight. You will pause for 1 second at the bottom of the lift. Then you'll take 1 second to lift the weight back up. Rest 10 seconds between sets.

Day 2 - Low-Volume

Perform the Day-2 low-volume routine 48 hours after the Day-1 high-volume routine.

Triple Drop Set Standing Calf Raises - Do 3 sets x 10-10-10 reps, respectively. You will perform 3 drop sets of 10 reps per drop set, for 30 total reps in each complete set. Each drop set will use a successively lower weight. Each rep is done at a 1-2-1 rhythm. Rest 90 seconds between sets.

Be sure to take the full 2-second pause at the bottom of the lift.

Given the intensity of these routines, be sure to stretch thoroughly.

. . .

Anti-Arnold Donkey Calf Raises

First of all, I am not Anti-Arnold. I love Arnold and especially his pioneering calf training. But Arnold is also known for loading several sweaty men onto his back for his donkey calf raises. I'm offering cleaner, less sweaty alternatives.

The magic of the donkey calf raise is that your calf muscles, particularly your gastrocnemius muscles, are forced into an ideal, fully stretched position at the bottom of the exercise. This fully stretched position makes you engage as many muscle fibers as possible when lifting.

Here are a few options for performing donkey calf raises:

1. If you don't have access to a donkey calf raise machine at your gym, strap on a loaded dipping belt and stand on a stable, elevated block with your toes on the edge of the block. Alternatively, use a Smith machine squat rack.
2. If using a dipping belt, bend at the waist, letting the weight hang between your legs. If using a Smith machine or donkey calf raise machine, bend at the waist, engage the weight on the bar, and let the weight rest—wherever it's comfortable—on your lower back, so that the weight drives directly down your legs.
3. Perform the donkey calf raises with your legs straight and the weight driving directly down through your legs and into your heels.
4. Make sure you are maximizing your range of movement. This means your feet will be traveling through a full range of motion with each repetition.
5. Your donkey calf raises can be performed in a bilateral or unilateral position with one or two legs. If using one leg, find something suitable to hold or rest on to maintain balance.
6. Use any rep ranges, weight setups, numbers of sets, contraction timing, or exercise variations required to fully fatigue your calves. See the *Variations* chapter for ideas.

For those working out at home, also think about donkey calf raises without summoning family members to sit on your back—if they're willing to help, then you're already good to go—all you need is a dog leash and dumbbells or weight plates.

Loop the leash around the dumbbell(s) or through the hole in the weight plate(s). Fasten the leash clamp around the leash's handle to make a loop. Step through the resulting loop, adjust the leash to rest around your hips, bend over, and let the weight hang between your legs. Now begin lifting!

Fascial Release and Other Recovery Techniques

If you're doing everything right and still not seeing the calf development you're after, you may want to try Active Release Therapy (ART) and similar massage programs.

Weight training and other demanding physical activities can lead to soft tissue damage over time. Tightness of the fascia—the supportive connective tissues surrounding your muscles, organs, bones, and blood vessels and which help hold them in place—may restrict muscle growth. Proper treatment of these damaged tissues with ART may help release these constraining tissues, allowing muscle growth to take place.

Here's one way to perform active release therapy for your calves on your own:

1. Sit on the floor or ground with one leg bent and the other straight.
2. On the elevated, bent leg, hold your calf with both hands. Place your thumbs on your shin with your fingers wrapped around your lower calf. While applying pressure with your hands, straighten your leg and flex your toes as your elevated leg comes to rest beside your supporting leg.

3. Return the formerly elevated leg to the starting position. Bend your leg and move your fingers up it to the middle of your calf. As before, apply pressure, and extend your leg with your toes pointed as you return it to the floor.
4. Repeat the same dynamic massage on the upper part of your calf.
5. Repeat the progressive massage on the inside and the outside of the muscle, starting from the bottom and working your way up, massaging the bottom, middle, and top portions of your calf as you extend your leg and point your toes.
6. Repeat the same procedure for the other leg.

Don't be limited to ART to help your body grow, release tension, and recover. Other techniques and approaches can provide positive recovery and preventative benefits such as:

1. Stretching, both dynamic and static.
2. Pressure, trigger point, and percussive self-massage.
3. Assisted massage—deep tissue, sports massage, shiatsu massage, lymphatic massage or reflexology.
4. Ice bath, cold water immersion or cold shower therapy.
5. Various relaxation, meditation, and visualization techniques.

HIIT Those Calves

High intensity training is generally considered to be training involving periods of exercise at or near maximal exertion followed by short periods of rest. These rest periods generally do not provide enough time for full recovery from the intense exertion.

Tabata training, for example, is one type of HIIT training method where you go through one or more exercises over a 4-minute period. Tabatas involve 8 x 20-second exertion phases and 8 x 10-second rest phases. So, over 4 minutes, you exert yourself at or near maximum effort for 20 seconds and then take a 10-second break 8 times in the 4-minute Tabata set.

Tabatas and HIIT can make great calf-building challenges. They allow you to put your calves through short, intense bursts of exertion. You could, for example, mix up as many calf exercises as you can think of in a single HIIT session or just focus on one.

One of my favorite HIIT sessions involves drop-set Tabatas with standing calf raises. If you don't have access to a calf-raise machine, use a weight vest or dumbbells as an alternative. After warming up for 20 seconds, perform normal single or double-legged calf raises with the maximum weight you can handle for 8 to 12 reps. When you can no longer lift that weight with good form, drop to a lower weight—during the rest cycles—and keep pushing in the active phases.

If your calves are not on fire after 8 successive sets with minimal rest between, you're not trying hard enough, not using enough weight, or using bad form.

HIIT training pushes you to your limits in short, intense time periods. As such, you may need significant recovery time after HIIT sessions. But your calves won't know what hit them.

The Challenge

This is a simple exercise intended to push your limits, much like the Mountain. This routine is also great incorporated into other programs or as a separate workout.

The Challenge is simple: perform as many single-leg calf raises as you can with each leg. Use good form controlling the motion—without bouncing—making sure to pause at the bottom and top of each rep. Use a step, a curb, a suitable rock, or anything else that will let you move through a complete motion. When you're unable to perform any more complete repetitions, continue with partial reps, performing partial contractions as high as you're able to press upward.

Finished with one leg? Then switch to the other. Set a goal and go for it! Once you've hit that goal, go for more!

As usual, consider intensifying the routine and throwing off your body's adaptations by increasing reps, slowing down reps, holding your stretch and contractions for longer at the bottom and top of your reps, adding weight, and any other variation that pushes you that bit further. As an alternative, perform the Challenge with both legs simultaneously instead of one leg at a time.

Climbing the Mountain

What happens when you cross The Challenge with The Mountain?

You climb the mountain!

Climbing the Mountain is another basic calf exercise challenge. Perform it doing either single or double-leg calf raises. Here's how Climbing the Mountain works. Find a set of stairs. If you don't have stairs, a single step —or sturdy object—will do, but you may lose some sense of accomplishment as you climb without visible upward movement and progress. Choose a number of reps to perform on each set, then climb away!

You'll do that number of repetitions on each step for each leg, individually or both at the same time. Once you've performed those repetitions, you go up to the next step.

Keep climbing, or repeating if you don't have access to stairs, until you have to stop and cannot climb any farther.

Choose whatever calf-raise variation(s) you want or change them as you climb—

extended peak contractions, extended calf stretches, explosive lifts, partial rep pauses, adding weight, extending the concentric and/or eccentric movement. Do whatever you can to challenge yourself and shock your muscles into growth as you move. Once you've reached your limits, remember how far you climbed and then try to surpass those limits the next time you climb the mountain!

As with the other approaches presented in *Killer Calves*, the important thing with these routines is to explore, experiment, and ultimately find what works for you. Once you've found what works, keep pushing to learn and do more.

Good luck and may the gains be with you!

WHAT'S NEXT?

The honest answer to that question is the next steps in your calf training and development are up to you. Just as you determine how hard you work and how much success you have, you will determine how much your calves grow and how well they are maintained.

Personally, I exercise my calves two to three times a day, every day. This is the level of commitment required for me to see results. Since I started working with this level of dedication, my calves—and I'm a hard gainer—have grown.

They are now larger than my biceps.

However, I know that if I stop exercising hard, varying my routines, and challenging myself, I will not see additional growth. I also know that if I do not work to maintain what I have gained, this progress will gradually disappear. With any luck, your road is much easier than mine.

But, whatever your journey, *Killer Calves* will get you there.

So, the choice is yours. *Killer Calves* offers you the tools needed to help you achieve the calves of your dreams, and hopefully the ideas presented here have inspired you to push and strive for your goals.

Remember, your calves, like your life, are what you make of them.

I want you to keep pushing, to never stop exploring, and to continually develop.

Then, your calves won't be the only thing that are killer.

—Rhys Larson

CITATIONS

Here are the sources for the quotes used in *Killer Calves*:

1. "The Complete Arnold: Calves." *Muscle & Fitness*, 9 June 2017, www.muscleandfitness.com/flexonline/training/complete-arnold-calves/.
2. "Lou Ferrigno's Mass Class." *Muscle & Fitness*, 29 Dec. 2015, www.muscleandfitness.com/flexonline/training/lou-ferrignos-mass-class/.
3. Old School Labs. *Secret to Historic Calves | Q&A with Golden Era Legend Tom Platz.* www.youtube.com/watch?v=yiJqIRoXVfk.
4. Ladon, Jacob. "This Mass Monster Has Some of the Craziest Monster Calves in Bodybuilding History." *Generation Iron Fitness & Bodybuilding Network,* 12 July 2019, generationiron.com/this-mass-monster-has-some-of-the-craziest-monster-calves-in-bodybuilding-history/.
5. "Want Calves Like Flex Lewis?" *Muscle & Fitness*, 19 July 2012, www.muscleandfitness.com/flexonline/training/want-calves-flex-lewis/.

BEASTLY

BICEPS

THE ESSENTIAL GUIDE TO BICEP GROWTH AND DEVELOPMENT

RHYS LARSON

PREFACE

A few words of caution and encouragement.

This book is about helping you reach your potential (and getting your biceps to grow).

Although pushing our limits helps us—and our biceps—grow and improve, we should exercise thoughtfully and with common sense.

As you work to build your biceps, don't take unnecessary risks or push yourself too hard, especially not to the point of injury.

Please consult a physician before embarking on any exercise program, especially if you have any questions or concerns about your body, your health, or your exercise limitations.

I want you exercising healthily.

It's the only way for those stubborn biceps to actually grow.

—Rhys Larson

BEASTLY BICEPS

Not everyone is born with the chiseled, well-muscled arms of their dreams. Whether you want arms that are bulging, defined, proportional, well-formed, massive, or shredded, *Beastly Biceps* can help make your dreams a reality.

For those who want to banish their underachieving arms to the distant past, *Beastly Biceps* will help turn your scrawny sticks into smoking guns.

For those who want to be fit, bring variety to their exercise routines, add upper arm development, or maintain what they have already worked so hard to attain, *Beastly Biceps* is for you too.

Beastly Biceps offers a broad range of tools, exercises, insights, and ideas to help shape and sculpt your arms, particularly your biceps.

So, if you're a hard gainer who has tried everything—or think you have —to build your biceps, *Beastly Biceps* will give you many novel ways to push your limits and help your muscles grow. If you're looking to sculpt and tone your arms, *Beastly Biceps* will provide you with a host of options to achieve the look you're after.

Or, if you're already jacked and looking to add a bit of variety and new options to your arm routines, *Beastly Biceps* will give you innovative ideas and programs to torture yourself both at home and in the gym.

Whether you're a fitness beginner looking for help, a seasoned bodybuilder or fitness professional looking for that little edge, someone who wants to get in shape, or an exercise enthusiast looking for new approaches and concepts, *Beastly Biceps* will help you improve your arms.

Everyone deserves a great pair of arms.

Everyone deserves a pair of beastly biceps!

HOW THIS BOOK WORKS

Beastly Biceps is built around the goal of giving you the tools and knowledge needed to get your biceps to develop and grow.

To do this, *Beastly Biceps* is broken into sections that will provide you numerous suggestions, background information, and a wide range of exercises and routines to try. The information ranges from basic exercises you may already know to crazy ideas you've never heard of, much less tried. These routines can be performed on their own or mixed in with other exercise programs to give you the best results possible. Added into your arm days, the exercises in *Beastly Biceps* will help more than just your biceps be beastly.

Beyond basic exercises and routines, *Beastly Biceps* will also offer numerous techniques and variations for each exercise to maximize growth and training effectiveness, as well as offering all the vital background information on how biceps work. I also include some basic anatomy to help you understand how to best achieve bicep development.

Finally—and this is a fundamental motivation for writing this book— by bringing all these ideas and approaches together in one place, I hope *Beastly Biceps* will inspire you to experiment, explore, and learn what approaches work best for you.

By learning what exercises and variations are most effective for you, I hope you will share your hard-earned knowledge and experience to help others boost their own arm game and reach all their individual fitness goals.

Whatever bicep targets you choose—whether it's massive biceps or sleek, well-proportioned arms—*Beastly Biceps* is here to make your goals possible.

BECOMING BICEP-DEDICATED

Training any lagging body part is not easy. If your biceps are not where you would like them or if they are stubbornly refusing to respond to your efforts, this frustration can lead to discouragement and interfere with your desire to reach your goals.

Although I cannot reach your goals for you, I *can* give you the tools to help you reach them. In turn, you *must* provide the motivation, the dedication, and the effort to bring those dreams to life. *Beastly Biceps* is also here to help ignite that spark.

Getting that fire to burn, to help you push through obstacles or disappointments and achieve the biceps of your dreams will take much work, however.

Yes, *lots* of work.

This process is not simple or quick.

But you can do it.

Beastly Biceps will give you all the tools to help your biceps grow, allowing you to overcome your deficiencies and stimulate only improvements.

But your dedication must fuel you to those goals. This is the part I cannot do for you.

You *must* be committed and put forth the necessary effort in spite of any setbacks or disappointments. You must generate your own enthusiasm and workout regime.

Simply going through the motions as you exercise, or breezing through workouts to pay lip service to them, will not get you where you want to be.

Your biceps look the way they do for a reason. They reflect the amount and type of effort you have put into them. So, if you haven't put in any work, or you haven't worked hard or effectively, then you haven't even scratched the surface of their growth potential.

Your job, your goal, is to counter your biceps' resistance to growth.

No amount of knowledge or range of exercises will do anything for you if you don't make your efforts and understanding count.

Beastly Biceps will get you started on your way to the arms of your dreams, but *you* are the one who has to get there… one curl at a time.

I ask you to train diligently, to persevere, and to embody your end goals with each and every rep. Push to reach your dreams because no one else will—or can—do it for you.

And then you, too, will have beastly biceps.

BICEP ANATOMY

If you want to build beastly biceps (or build up your biceps at all), you need to understand your muscle anatomy. This way, you'll know precisely what muscles to target, recognize how to target them, and understand how to work toward your bicep goals.

This is not to say that you won't be able to build your biceps if you don't know your anatomy—because you can and will—but rather, this means that you can help your biceps grow and develop more effectively and efficiently if you do.

Trial and error works but this approach can also be trialing, with lots of errors!

Trial with fewer errors is better.

Understanding so you can perform the *most effective* trials works best.

I want to help you avoid those trials, prevent those errors, and avoid the pitfalls that will interfere with achieving your goals.

Your upper arm is located between the elbow and shoulder joints and contains four major muscles. The three muscles in the front of the upper arm—also known as the anterior compartment—are the biceps brachii, the brachialis, and the coracobrachialis.

Together, these three muscles make up the bicep.

The triceps brachii—or triceps—is on the back or posterior of the arm—also known as the posterior compartment—and is composed of three heads —the medial, lateral, and long heads. Taken together, these four muscle groups comprise the upper arm.

Without going into too much additional detail, the biceps brachii is a two-headed muscle consisting of a long and short head that flexes the arm at the elbow and shoulder—what most people think of as the bicep—and is involved in supination of the forearm.

The biceps brachii also flexes the arm at the elbow and at the shoulder, and contributes to the bicep peak toward which most people are aiming when working their arms.

The coracobrachialis muscle lies beneath the biceps brachii and aids in flexion of the arm at the shoulder and weak adduction—movement of the arm away from the body.

The coracobrachialis may well be the smallest muscle of the upper arm, but it helps adds fullness to the upper portion of the bicep.

Similarly, the brachialis muscle also lies beneath the biceps brachii and is responsible for flexion at the elbow joint—exercises such as hammer curls engage the brachialis. The brachialis muscle helps provide separation between the bicep and triceps while also contributing to the peak of the bicep by adding volume below the biceps brachii.

Most bicep exercises focus on the twin-headed biceps brachii but development of all upper arm muscles—especially the brachialis in conjunction with the biceps brachii—plays a major role in visible bicep muscle development. Throughout *Beastly Biceps*, I will share a variety of exercises and routines to help you to develop all aspects of your bicep muscles.

BICEP EXERCISES

You may go to the gym to get ripped, to add mass, to get in shape to be able to do what you love, to build tree-trunk legs, develop a perfect v-taper, sculpt boulder shoulders, to create a chiseled physique, or lose some weight.

Or you may go for something entirely different. However, one of the most attainable fitness goals for many gym goers is well-developed arms, particularly the biceps.

The biceps may not be the biggest muscles in your arms—the triceps have that distinction—but they are often the most noticeable, and biceps are what many people think of when they think of muscular arms. In this chapter, I'll give you an overview of some of the most common bicep exercises to get those biceps bulging, and the form required to get them growing.

Standing Curls

Standing curls are a true bicep classic and one of the foundational bicep exercises.

Standing bicep curls can be performed with dumbbells, kettlebells, or exercise bands. Each different piece of equipment brings slight variations and challenges to the lift to help your bicep development.

To perform standing curls, get a pair of dumbbells and let them hang at arm's length next to your thighs. Rotate your arms so that your palms face forward. Holding your upper arms locked in position, bend your elbows as you lift, curling the dumbbells straight upward, and lifting up as close to your shoulders as possible.

Hold the weight at the top, focusing on the bicep peak, then slowly lower the weight back down to the starting position. You can easily add variety to standing curls by lifting upward outside or inside the plane of your body, in addition to straight up.

The lifting motion is similar for both kettlebells and exercise bands as well. With bands, varying your foot placement and band length will adjust the tension. With kettlebells, racking the weight so that it rests on the back of your forearms can help with stability.

Standing Barbell Curls

To do standing barbell curls, after adding your desired weight, pick up the barbell with an underhand grip, bringing the bar to your waist. Position your hands at roughly hip width and vary your hand placement to change the exercise focus.

For example, use a wider grip to hit the inner head of the bicep.

Use a narrower grip to target the outer portion of the bicep.

Begin your exercise with the bar at hip height. Tighten your core as you begin the lift and contract your biceps as you curl the bar up to shoulder height. To add additional emphasis on the biceps, squeeze at the top of the movement. After contracting, slowly lower the weight back down to the starting position at your waist. Control the weight throughout the exercise but especially on the downward eccentric movement. For stability, keep your core engaged and your feet planted throughout the exercise. To main-tain the focus on your biceps, do not rock, swing, or use your hips to help lift the weight.

. . .

Standing Hammer Curls

Standing hammer curls can be performed with dumbbells, kettlebells, or exercise bands. Each different piece of equipment brings slight variations and challenges to the lift.

Select a pair of dumbbells—or kettlebells or an exercise band—and let the weight hang by your sides at arm's length.

Your palms will face inward toward your thighs throughout the exercise. Holding your upper arms in place, bend your elbows and lift, curling the dumbbells up as close to your shoulders as possible. Pause, holding the biceps tight at the top of the curl, and then slowly lower the weight back to the starting position by your thighs.

The lifting motion is similar for both kettlebells and exercise bands as well. With bands, varying your foot placement and band length will adjust the tension. With kettlebells, racking the weight so that it rests on the back of your forearms can help with stability.

Alternative Hammer Curls—Cable or Towel Curls

As an alternative to more traditional hammer curls with weights, hammer curls can also be performed using a rope on the low pulley of a cable machine or with a towel or rope looped through or around weights or kettlebells. Like hammer curls with bands, hammer curls with a towel, rope, or cable provide a bit more flexibility through the curling movement to help hit the biceps from slightly different angles.

To begin, attach a rope to the cable pulley machine or loop a towel or rope through the handle of a weight or kettlebell. Grip the rope or towel firmly, holding with your palms facing inward in a neutral position, like you would use for a traditional hammer curl with dumbbells. For stability, engage your posterior chain and core to create a stable foundation, and then lift, squeezing your biceps as you bring the rope or towel up as high as possible. Hold the contraction at the top of the lift before lowering your hands back down by your waist. Keep your body stable to avoid using any momentum as you curl.

EZ Bar Preacher Curls

The preacher curl takes its name from the kneeling position employed while doing lifts. The exercise works best with a declined preacher bench, but you can be creative and use other objects such as an exercise ball or the arms of a couch if you're working out at home.

Load up an EZ bar with your desired weights and place your hands six inches apart; as with other curls, you can vary the spacing between your hands to change the exercise's emphasis. Taking position at the preacher bench, rest your triceps on the sloping pad of the preacher bench. Hold the EZ bar in front of you with your arms not quite straight—you'll want to maintain a slight bend in the elbows. Holding your upper arms still on the pad, lift the weight upward from your wrists, bending your arms at the elbow as you curl the bar toward your shoulders. Pause at the top of the lift. Slowly lower the weight back to the starting position after your contraction at the top.

As an alternative, this lift can also be performed with a barbell. A further variation, referred to as a Scott curl, is performed similarly. However, with the Scott curl, your armpits and chest are both resting completely against the preacher bench pads. This strictly controlled motion isolates the exercise almost entirely in your biceps since you cannot generate momentum from your torso, shoulder, or hips.

Dumbbell Preacher Curls

This exercise utilizes the preacher bench just like the EZ bar preacher curls, except you're lifting dumbbells instead of the EZ bar. The preacher bench can also be used with a straight barbell or exercise bands. Dumbbell preacher curls allow you to perform the exercise with one arm, if desired, to really concentrate on the bicep one arm at a time.

As with the EZ bar preacher curls, begin by placing your upper arm(s) on the bench. Holding the dumbbell or dumbbells in place, trying to leave as little space between the back of your arm and the top of the bench as possible.

Do your best to keep the back of your upper arm on the bench throughout the exercise.

To avoid using momentum to cheat, tighten your core and buttocks as you sit and begin curling. Squeeze your biceps to lift the dumbbell(s) up, pausing to hold the contraction at the top of the curl. Maintain constant tension by placing your mind in the muscle and holding that exertion throughout each repetition.

Machine Preacher Curls

This exercise utilizes a preacher curl machine with a built-in bench instead of dumbbells or the EZ bar. Machine preacher curls allow you to perform the exercise with one arm, if desired, to really concentrate your effort.

To add a further variation, perform your one-armed machine preacher curls with an open palm, leaving your bicep and shoulder to take the majority of the load.

As with the other preacher curls, begin by placing your upper arm(s) on the bench. Holding the handle or handles in place, try to leave as little space between the back of your arm and the top of the bench. Do your best to keep the back of your upper arm on the bench throughout the exercise. To avoid using momentum to cheat, tighten your core and buttocks as you sit and begin curling. Squeeze your biceps to lift the handle(s) up, pausing to hold the contraction at the top of the curl. Maintain constant tension by placing your attention in the muscle as you work, and hold that exertion throughout each repetition.

Lying Preacher Curls

. . .

Lying preacher curls are not meant to imply or be confused with an untruthful preacher! These are, of course, preacher curls performed on your back while you're lying on a bench or the ground. These can be performed with a cable pull-down station or with bands affixed to a stationary object.

Position the bench—or your body on the floor—beneath the cable or band. Make sure your head is in line with the bar attached to the cable or bands when you lie down. Reach straight up to grab the bar, and, keeping your upper arms stationary, bend your elbows and squeeze your biceps as you curl the bar toward your head. To give additional emphasis to the bicep, you also can rotate your upper arms toward your head as you reach peak bicep contraction, and squeeze. As you curl, keep your shoulders still and your body stable to emphasize the bicep contraction at the bottom of the movement when the bar approaches your head. Release the contraction and control the weight on the way back.

Concentration Curls

The concentration curl is performed seated with your arm hanging between your legs.

As you lift the weight upward, your elbow will remain braced on your inner thigh just above the knee.

To do your concentration curls, you'll need a dumbbell and a chair or bench.

Sit on the chair or bench and spread your legs wide enough to allow space for your arm to curl as you lift the bicep.

For stability, rest your non-working arm on your thigh opposite to your working arm.

Let your arm hang down vertically with the elbow of your lifting arm resting on the same side leg, just above the knee on the inner thigh, toward your groin. As you begin the lift, keep your core firm and your torso upright by stabilizing your body with your off hand or elbow resting on your thigh. Curl the weight up, controlling through the lift.

Put your mind in the muscle, making sure to squeeze the bicep throughout exertion. Pause at the top of the lift and then lower the weight back into the starting position.

Spider Curls

Spider curls are performed leaning forward on an incline bench or chair with the weight hanging downward directly from your shoulders. Having your torso resting on the bench—or a padded chair if you're being creative and working out at home—will minimize cheating and focus the work to your bicep. With the spider curl, you'll be lifting diagonally across your body. Because you cannot engage the rest of your body to lift, you'll probably want to use a lighter weight than normal for your spider curls.

To perform your spider curls, get a dumbbell—or dumbbells if you want to do both arms at once, taking turns as you lift with each arm—and sit facing forward on an incline bench. Lean forward and rest your weight fully on the bench. With your arm hanging down as you lean forward, keeping your arm vertical and moving only at the elbow, squeeze your bicep to curl the dumbbell upward toward your shoulders, maintaining good form throughout the lift. As an alternative variation, curl the dumbbell diagonally across your body or use a barbell or EZ bar. For extra difficulty, pause and contract your bicep at the top of the lift. Keep your back engaged to prevent your shoulders from interfering with the movement, and focus on working the muscle throughout the entirety of the lift.

Decline Dumbbell Curls

Much like spider curls, decline dumbbell curls are performed leaning forward on an incline bench or chair with the weights hanging downward from your shoulders. Unlike spider curls, however, in decline dumbbell curls, you'll be lifting straight up and not diagonally.

Having your torso resting on the bench—or a padded chair if you're being creative and working out at home with minimal equipment—will minimize cheating and focus the work on your bicep. Because you cannot engage the rest of your body to lift, you'll probably want to use a lighter weight than with standing curls.

To perform your decline dumbbell curls, get a pair of dumbbells and lie with your chest resting against a bench set to a 45-degree angle. Let the weights hang down directly from your shoulders as you prepare to lift. Holding your upper arms in place, bend your elbows and curl the dumbbells straight up to your shoulders getting as close to your shoulders with the weight as you can. Hold the weight at the top, flexing your bicep, and then lower the weight to the starting position with full control throughout the motion. You can change arm angles and hand grips to add variation, as well going from a more traditional curl to a hammer curl—and beyond to a Zottman curl, detailed a few paragraphs below—with your palms facing down toward the ground.

Incline Dumbbell Curls

Much like decline curls, incline dumbbell curls are performed leaning on an incline bench or chair with the weights hanging downward from your shoulders. With inline dumbbell curls, however, you will be leaning backward with your back resting against the bench as your curl. Having your torso resting on the bench—or a padded chair if you're working out at home and don't have a bench—will minimize cheating and focus the work on your bicep.

To perform incline dumbbell curls, get a pair of dumbbells and lie with your back resting against a bench set to a 45-degree angle. With the weights hanging down from your shoulders and slightly behind you, keep your upper arms stationary, bend your elbows, and curl the dumbbells upward, bringing them as close to your shoulders as possible.

Hold the contraction at the top of the lift, then lower the weight back with full control to the starting position of the exercise. As with the decline dumbbell curls, you can change grip position and arm angles to add variation.

Zottman Curls

Aside from having one of the absolute best names for a bicep exercise, Zottman curls—named after George Zottman, an American strongman from Philadelphia who used to curl fifty pounds this way—also hit every major muscle head of the bicep by rotating from an underhand to an overhand grip halfway through the exercise.

To perform Zottman curls, select a pair of dumbbells and let the weight hang at arm's length next to your sides. Rotate your arms so that your palms face forward. Keeping your upper arms stationary and your core tight to minimize cheating, curl the dumbbells up, bringing the weight as close to your shoulders as you can.

Hold the weight at the top of the contraction as you flex.

Now rotate the dumbbells so that your palms face forward again before lowering. Keeping your hands in that position, slowly lower the weights to your sides with your knuckles remaining up. Rotate the dumbbells back around to the starting position, and repeat.

Waiter's Curls

The waiter's curl—so named because, throughout your curl, you're trying to keep the top of the dumbbell flat and in line with the floor like a waiter holds drinks stable on a tray—is performed using a single dumbbell and is a great way to add peaks to your biceps.

To perform the waiter's curl, start in a standing position with a single dumbbell centered in front of you, similar to the starting position in a goblin squat.

Hold the top of the dumbbell—beneath one head or weight plate—with one hand on either side. Your palms will be facing up under each side of the dumbbell throughout the exercise, which means your wrists will flex through the curl. To help with proper form, as you curl the weight up, imagine that the top of the dumbbell has a drink on it—one you get to drink after you're done!—that you do not want to spill.

Be sure to keep your shoulders stable to prevent engagement in the curl.

Coupled with not curling the wrists, not engaging the shoulders will concentrate the work on the biceps. This intense, controlled motion will encourage strong peak contractions and bigger heads on your biceps.

Combining the Spider Curl with the Waiter's Curl creates a supervillain-worthy combo—*the Spider Waiter!*—that will blast your biceps to the heavens. For this bicep combination, lean forward and let your arms hang on an incline bench as if you were performing a spider curl, but lift a single weight with both hands using the waiter's technique where the top of the weight remains parallel to the floor and your wrists flex through the curl to keep the weight flat.

Cheat Curls

Cheat curls are performed much like a normal standing curl, except you're lifting heavier weight than normal through an incomplete motion or partial rep, using the momentum of your hips and body to drive the weight upward.

Select the heaviest dumbbells that you can handle in a standing curl. Curl the weight up as you would for a conventional dumbbell curl. Use momentum from your hips to drive through the lift and overcome the point of most difficulty halfway up the curl.

You are not flinging the weights up, however.

You are using momentum to assist in lifting a weight that you might not otherwise be able to handle for multiple reps. As you lift, do not lean back. Instead, you'll need to find a rhythm where you rock your torso forward and back while extending your hips to complete each rep.

Although you're 'cheating', cheat curls are meant to be challenging, not easy. Push to your limits, to within a rep of your maximum.

Drag Curls

Drag curls use a motion similar to an upright row(e.g., lifting the weight(s) up leading with your elbows), except you're standing straight up and using dumbbells—you can use a bar as an alternative—as you curl. You're also not curling the dumbbells up from your hands. Instead, you're lifting with your elbows as the dumbbells slide along your sides.

To perform a drag curl, pick up a pair of dumbbells and bring them up beside your hips as the weight hangs by your sides—the standard starting position for a standing bicep curl. As you begin the lift, stand tall while you drive your elbows back and up as you curl. Keep your palms facing up and forward during the lift. As you lift, the inside head of each dumbbell will remain in contact with the side of your body throughout the curl. As you curl, you are dragging the weights up and down along the sides of your hips and chest. If performed with a bar, the bar will drag along the front of your stomach and chest as you lift up from your waist toward your shoulders.

Hanging Inverted Rows

Inverted rows are performed with your upper body hanging at an angle suspended from a bar, your heels resting on the ground away from you for stability. Your hands can be placed overhand, underhand, or split between over- and underhand grips. Inverted rows are an assisted pullup variation.

To keep the emphasis on your arms as much as possible, lock your back in place and try to lift with your arms as much as you can.

Grab onto a bar with an underhand, overhand, or mixed shoulder-width grip. Depending on your grip, your palms will be facing toward or away from you.

Hang from the bar with your arms completely straight, with your heels resting on the ground at full body length away—bringing your feet closer to your hands will take some weight off your arms. In this position, your body should form a straight line from your feet to your head. Begin by pulling your shoulders back, holding the shoulder blades in place. Pull with your arms—not your back—to lift your chest up to the bar. Hold at the top and then lower your body back down to the starting position in a stable, controlled motion. Variations of the inverted row can also be performed on gymnastic rings, using ropes, via bands, or using suspension training systems.

Chin-ups

Unlike many other bicep exercises that really focus on isolating the work on the biceps, the chin-up recruits other muscles during the exertion. The degree to which your biceps work is strongly influenced by how much you engage your back during the lift.

Using a shoulder-width underhand grip, grab a chin-up bar and hang at arm's length. To minimize back engagement, squeeze your shoulder blades down and back and focus on lifting with your arms. Bend your arms at the elbows and pull your chest toward the bar, touching it if possible. Hold at the top, squeezing your biceps, and then slowly lower your body back down to the starting position. Don't drop...keep the tension focused in your biceps as you lower. To add variety, bring your arms closer together, spread them wider apart, add weight, or even work toward one-armed chin-ups.

Bent-Over Barbell Rows

Bent-over barbell rows are the standing equivalent of the hanging inverted row.

Instead of pulling yourself up to the bar to lift, you will pull a bar up toward your body in bent-over rows. Just as with hanging inverted rows, you can vary your hand positions and widths to change the lift emphasis.

To start, pick up a barbell with your hands placed just outside shoulder-width apart. Hold the bar at arm's length and bend forward at your hips and knees—almost like you're starting a Romanian deadlift. Tighten your core and posterior chain to lock your body into position. As you lift, pull the bar upward to your ribcage. Hold at the top of the lift, contracting your biceps, and then lower the bar back down to the starting position.

Seated Cable Rows

Like chin-ups and bent-over barbell rows, seated cable rows take advantage of potential back exercises and turn them into bicep blasters.

To perform seated cable rows, take a seat on a bench or chair at a seated cable row station—if you're exercising at home, bands can be used as well. Place your feet firmly on the platform and let your knees bend slightly. As you prepare to pull, hold a V-bar or handle with your palms facing one another. To minimize ancillary muscle recruitment, hold your stomach tight, maintain a flat back, do not engage or pull with your back, hips, and legs, and draw your shoulders back as you pull the bar toward your torso.

Kneeling Single- or Double-Armed Curls

Pick up a pair of dumbbells and kneel down—if you have knee issues, a soft mat or other cushioned surface can help here. For stability, you can rest on one knee and keep your other leg bent with your foot resting on the ground. Hold one of the dumbbells relaxed by your side with your palm facing inward, toward your thigh. Keeping your upper arm stationary, bend your elbow as you lift and curl the dumbbell upward, rotating your arm as you lift.

Bring the dumbbell as close to your shoulder as you can. Hold the weight at the top, maintaining a peak contraction and then lower the weight down to the starting position.

Perform all the repetitions on your one arm before switching to the other. Alternatively, you can switch between arms with each rep. For variations, you can change hand positions, lift types, or use different weights—EZ bar, bands, or other weights.

Racked Farmer's Carry—and Other Isometric Holds

The farmer's carry is another exercise not generally thought of as a bicep exercise.

In fact, the farmer's carry—racked or not—is a whole-body exercise.

However, by holding your arms locked in place as you walk—or stand in place—the isometric exercise will do wonders for your biceps.

To perform a racked farmer's carry, pick up a pair of dumbbells and lift them up into the racked position so that each dumbbell is above your shoulders, the back of the dumbbell directly *above* your shoulders, by the side of your head. Holding the weights in place, walk forward for ten meters or yards, turn around, and then walk back. To increase difficulty, you can adjust where you hold the weight as you walk. Racked farmer's carries are one of many isometric biceps holds you can perform. You can perform isometric holds for any bicep exercise and even incorporate them into your lifts. Adding an isometric hold during the middle of a lift adds a bit of glorious muscle-building torture to your bicep routine.

Cable Flex Curls or Standing Band Curls

Cable flex curls can be performed one arm at a time or using both simultaneously, depending on what works best for you. The single-arm version lends the exercise additional stability, core work, and focus.

To perform your cable flex curls, position yourself in the middle of the weight stacks of a cable crossover station. Take in hand a handle from the high pulley location on each side. Hold your arms out to the sides at about shoulder height, so they're parallel to the floor—imagine yourself as Samson if you want to channel your inner power but just don't bring the gym down with the biceps you'll develop! Holding your right arm stationary, curl your left hand toward your head and hold the contraction.

Allow your left arm to straighten and then repeat the move with your right. Alternatively, bring in both arms at the same time. Either way, maintain stability and control throughout the movement, keeping a good foundation as you curl.

Standing flex curls can also be performed with bands anchored about shoulder height using a similar motion.

Behind-the-Back Cable Curls

Behind-the-back cable curls are a variation of the standard seated or standing cable curl. However, instead of curling within a standard curl range (i.e., from the waist up to the shoulder), you'll be curling up from behind your hip and up to your shoulder.

To perform behind-the-back cable curls, first attach a D-handle to the low pulley of a cable machine. Take the handle in one hand and step away from the machine, leaving the arm holding the cable handle straight and slightly behind your body.

This starting position will put tension on the cable and your arm as you begin.

Stagger your feet for stability (e.g., bring the opposite foot from your working arm forward). Curl the handle up toward your shoulder as high as possible, but don't let your elbow move forward while you hold your upper arm in place. Contract and hold at the top of the curl and feel the exertion in your bicep. Lower the handle back down to the starting position, keeping your arm stable and extended before beginning the next rep.

Switch sides when done. Alternately, curl both arms simultaneously while keeping your torso and upper arms stable.

~

These are a few of the many bicep exercises you can and will see used throughout *Beastly Biceps*. There are many others, including ones you may come up with yourself.

Coupled with variations for each exercise, and combining the exercises in novel routines, you'll have a lifetime to explore ways to torture your biceps.

Whatever exercises and variations you use, maintain good form and keep working for those gains! Bulging biceps will soon be your reward!

COMPOUND CURLS

Bicep curls are often simple exercises that focus on isolating the bicep muscles.

But they don't have to be.

With *Beastly Biceps*, I want to show you other techniques to work your biceps, ways to challenge yourself—and your muscles—in new and interesting ways. Compound curls—bicep exercises that incorporate multiple muscle groups and joint movements—are one way to engage your body more fully while still blasting and building your biceps.

Here are some non-traditional bicep exercises that engage more than just your biceps:

Kneeling Single-Arm Curl

Your biceps have two primary functions: to bend your elbows, and to rotate—supinate—your forearms. Working both bending and rotating functions of your biceps with heavy weights and low reps leads to rapid results in your arms. Curling from a kneeling position, with the weight focused on one side of your body, will challenge your obliques and other stability muscles to keep you upright and work your core and biceps simultaneously.

Here's how:

Choose a dumbbell you can curl for no more than 5 reps or curl no longer than 15 seconds. Hold the dumbbell in your off—nondominant—hand, palm facing inward, and kneel. Keeping your elbow against your ribs, curl the weight, twisting your hand so that your palm faces your shoulder at the top of the curl. Perform 3 reps on each side, alternating back and forth between your right and left hands as many times as you can in five minutes.

Once you can go back and forth 10 times (for a total of 30 reps on each side), in a single session, increase the weight.

Deep Swimmer's Press

The deep swimmer's press combines the biceps curl and the shoulder press into one complex, arm- and shoulder-building movement. With the deep swimmer's press, you'll work all the major muscles in your upper arms with just one exercise, making this an especially great exercise if you are looking to add variety to your arm workouts or want to make your weight training sessions more efficient.

Here's how:

Generally, the deep swimmer's press is performed from a standing position, but it can also be performed while sitting or kneeling. Start by holding a pair of dumbbells down by your sides, with your palms facing forward and your elbows pointing behind you as if you were going to perform a standard bicep curl. Begin curling by bending your elbows and lifting the dumbbells up to your shoulders. Your elbows should be directly in-line underneath your wrists, with your palms facing your shoulders. From this mid-way position, press the weights overhead, twisting your wrists 180 degrees as you push up so that your palms finish facing forward when your arms are fully extended.

To complete the movement, lower the dumbbells back to your shoulders, rotating your wrists so that your palms face your shoulders again, and then extend your elbows and lower the dumbbells to return the weights back to the starting position by your sides.

As an alternative, perform the deep swimmer's press using one arm at a time.

For an intensifier, hold the non-pressing arm at ninety degrees—keep your forearm parallel to the ground—with a dumbbell in hand for an isometric bicep exercise while your other arm works.

Arnold's Press Curl

The Arnold's Press is a classic whole-shoulder exercise involving shoulder rotation, while lifting up into a press from the starting position with dumbbells, kettlebells, or bands held together in front of the chest. When combined with a bicep curl to start and finish the movement, the Arnold's press will blast your gains into the stratosphere. As a complete arm exercise, use the Arnold's press curl to add efficiency and variety to your arm workouts.

Here's how:

As with the swimmer's press, the Arnold's press is performed from a standing position, but can also be performed sitting or kneeling. Start by holding a pair of dumbbells down by your sides with your palms facing forward and your elbows pointing behind you as if you were going to perform a standard bicep curl. Begin curling by bending your elbows and lifting the dumbbells up to a racked position in front of your upper chest.

Your elbows should be directly in-line underneath your wrists, with your palms facing your shoulders. From this mid-way position, press the weights overhead, but do not push straight up. Instead, rotate your elbows outward and your arms around and behind in a semicircle as you press up. Twist your wrists 180 degrees as you push up, so that your palms finish facing forward when your arms are fully extended at the top of the press.

To complete the movement, lower the dumbbells back to your shoulders, making another half-circle with your arms as you control the weight down, rotating your wrists so that your palms face your shoulders again.

Then extend your elbows and lower the dumbbells through the bottom half of the curl to return the weights back to the starting position by your sides.

As an alternative, perform the Arnold's press curl using one arm at a time.

For an intensifier, hold the non-pressing arm at ninety degrees—keep your forearm parallel to the ground and the weight locked in place—with a dumbbell in hand for an isometric bicep exercise while your other arm works.

For additional variety and intensity, adjust your tempo, add pauses, increase the weight, add reps, or use any other variation that works your biceps and shoulders effectively.

Split-jack Curl

Using lighter weights, the split-jack curl makes a solid cardio exercise that also works your biceps. Using heavier weights, the split-jack curl becomes an intense power-training exercise. The deeper you sink into a lunge and the faster you jump out of it, the more you target your fast-twitch muscle fibers as you exercise.

Here's how:

. . .

Hold a pair of dumbbells by your sides, with your palms facing inward, and your feet hip-width apart. Jump into a split stance—starting with either leg forward—while simultaneously curling the weights to your shoulders. Return to the starting position and repeat, landing with your opposite leg forward. Continue alternating split jumps and curling for 20 seconds or 10 reps. To make the exercise more challenging, drop into a full lunge as you land. For a quick, 4-minute cardio bicep-focused workout, rest 10 seconds after each set and do 8 sets—or as many as you can manage while maintaining good form.

Squat Concentration Curl

Squat concentration curls force your thighs outward and help open up your hips while you work your biceps. Pressing your upper arms against your thighs isolates the curling movement at your elbows, preventing other muscles from assisting. Squat concentration curls give you a great arm workout, while countering the mobility loss caused by far too much sitting in our normal day-to-day lives.

Here's how:

Pick up a pair of light dumbbells (e.g., 10 to 15 pounds), stand with your feet roughly shoulder-width apart, and point your toes slightly outward. Push your hips back and squat down until your thighs are parallel to the floor. While keeping your weight balanced on your heels, your elbows pressed against your inner thighs, and your palms facing one another, curl the weights for 30 to 60-seconds.

Maintain good form while you curl the weight up and down.

For additional instability and to increase the challenge to your core, curl one arm at a time.

. . .

Plank Curl or Push-up Position Hammer Curl

This exercise is reminiscent of a row performed in a plank or pushup position—a plank row. But, instead of pulling the dumbbell up by your side to do a row, you'll do a curl instead. Doing a curl instead of a row moves the exercise load farther away from your center of gravity and base of support. As a result, your core muscles need to work harder to stabilize your spine, making this one of the best ab exercises you probably didn't even know about.

Here's how:

Place a pair of dumbbells on the floor and assume a push-up position with your palms facing each other. Without moving your upper arm, curl the weight in your left hand toward your left shoulder. Lower it and repeat with your right arm. Continue alternating between left and right curls for 30 to 60-seconds. As you get stronger, add weight but speed up the movement. As an alternative, instead of performing hammer curls in your plank position, try curling across your body for a standard curl.

Resistance Band Jumping-jack Hammer Curl

Resistance band jumping-jack hammer curls are a fun way to work your biceps and send your heart rate soaring. Jumping against bands also targets the hip muscles that provide stability during lunges and squats... muscles that are rarely worked directly. Strengthening these hip stability muscles can improve the appearance of your lower body, help protect your knees and back, and work your biceps as well.

. . .

Here's how:

Stand with your feet together, centered on top of a looped resistance band. Hold the top of the band with your palms facing each other for a hammer-type curl or toward the ceiling for a traditional curl. Curl the band toward your shoulders and jump outward with both feet—your feet move through a standard jumping-jack as you curl.

Reverse the move to return to the starting position. Repeat the exercise for 20 seconds or 10 total reps. Do 8 sets, resting for 10 seconds between each set.

Add variety by alternating sets of curls and overhead presses (e.g., 4 sets of each), changing curl type, switching to jumping squats instead of jumping jacks, adding more resistance, increasing your number of sets or exercise time. Consider gloves if the bands abrade your skin while stretching and contracting.

These are just a few of many complex, multi-joint exercises that can be performed while working your biceps. Go out, discover more, and get those biceps bulging!

EXERCISE VARIATIONS

Beastly Biceps is filled with different exercises and approaches to develop your biceps. But one thing I need to stress is that you will ultimately have to find out what works best for you to achieve your bicep goals. Whatever exercises and techniques you try, you will need to be patient, persistent, maximize your effort, listen to your body, and, above all else, be willing to push your boundaries to achieve your dreams.

Every exercise and exercise routine in *Beastly Biceps* can be modified and adapted to help you grow and push your limits. Think of yourself as a mad (or not so mad... infinitely sane, if you prefer) fitness scientist searching out the best ways to unlock your growth and development potential.

This process takes work and quite a bit of creativity.

Use this opportunity, your focused effort, and your ingenuity to your advantage to help yourself grow! So, as you try out the routines, exercises, and ideas in *Beastly Biceps,* here are some variations you can use on almost any exercise to push your limits, overcome boredom and muscle adaptation, and build those biceps!

Ways to vary almost any exercise include:

1. **Reps** – Vary the number of repetitions required to push your limits. As your strength and endurance grow, you can increase the weight you push and/or the number of repetitions performed.
2. **Sets** – Like reps, increasing or decreasing the numbers of sets for a given exercise is always an option for bicep development whether your focus is on mass or definition.
3. **Time under tension** – Vary the time working, the time spent moving through the exercise, the time held contracting the bicep at the top of the raise, the time lowering the weight, and/or the time relaxed at the bottom of the motion to reduce or extend the time of your physical exertion. You can also adjust the length and rate of time spent in the concentric—contraction—or eccentric—lengthening or extension—phases of your exercises.
4. **Weight** – Adding or subtracting weight is one of the classic ways to vary exercises. Not only can you add or subtract weight as you work through your sets, but you can also do the same within a set (e.g., drop sets or reverse drop sets). This will allow you to not only increase your total load (the amount of weight lifted in a given set) but can also extend your time under tension as you fight against muscle failure (such as when performing drop sets) to facilitate muscle growth.
5. **Explosivity / Intensity**– Adjust the amount of energy or plyometric activation you put into each exercise. For instance, explode upward during the bicep raise and then go down slowly, accelerate through your lift starting slowly and gradually build speed as you elevate, or really exert yourself during your lift to maximize muscle engagement and get that burning pump.
6. **Join the chain gang** – Add chains or bands to your lifts to add intensity and increase resistance throughout the motion. Adding chains or bands is particularly effective in lifts involving bars like barbells but also works for dumbbells and other exercises. Bands and chains also change the amount of strength required in different portions of the exercise (e.g., by adding progressive resistance and the amount of muscle engagement to the lift).
7. **Change how you move through the exercise** – Employ

continuous and discontinuous movements to shock your biceps. For example, include pulses at the top of your bicep raise while holding the weight at full muscle contraction or muscular extension. Or include pauses or holds during the middle of the motion.

8. **Exercise orientation** – Shift the orientation of your hands and the primary focus of the exercise during an exercise. For instance, classic examples include rotating your hands outward, pointing your fingers in, squeezing the bar, or bending your wrists during exercise.

9. **Change stress and strain direction** – Shift where the exercise tension moves through your biceps by changing where the exertion moves through your arms when you lift. For example, curling up and rotating from little fingers instead of lifting straight up or rotating the weight inward from the outside of your hand.

10. **Adjust the orientation of your bodyweight** – During exercise, adjust your body's angle to shift how the weight and exercise tension move through your muscles. For instance, you can lean forward, backward, sideways, adjust your shoulder and back tension, or stay centered during the exercise to increase intensity and alter the focus of exertion.

11. **Adjust the smoothness or continuity of your motions** – Although we tend to move fluidly through an exercise with continuity of motion, we can also change this to shock our muscles. Instead of completing the whole movement in one smooth motion, we can break it down into sections, each with different movement patterns.

12. **Surprise to overcome adaptation** – Change your routines to continue pushing your development. If your biceps have adapted to your routine, their growth will suffer. A simple way to evaluate whether your biceps have adapted to your routine is if they are no longer sore the day after you work out. If your biceps aren't sore, consider changing your routine or increasing your intensity during your workouts. If you haven't shocked

your biceps to the point of soreness, they might not respond as well as you would like with growth.

13. **Workout with a partner** – While not an exercise variation per se, working out with a partner can vary and intensify your routine, open up new exercise options, and give you ideas for new exercises. Finding someone to exercise with can help motivate you, inspire you, and get you to the gym. When you're there, your partner can help push your limits and offer advice, particularly on issues you might otherwise miss. These opportunities coupled with your partner's encouragement can be the key to untapped gains. A partner can spot you to keep you safe, assist you so that you can lift more and longer than you thought possible, and, most importantly, a partner can help make your workouts more fun.

14. **Create inefficiencies** – Create inefficiencies in your movements. Sometimes, good form isn't enough to get your muscles to grow. Creating inefficiencies in your exercises makes the muscles you are targeting work harder to go through the movement. Creating inefficiency is *not* advocating using bad form when you exercise. Creating inefficiencies is another way of saying doing your reps using only—at least, as much as possible—the muscles targeted by a given lift to perform the exercise. For example, when doing bicep curls, your body tends to move efficiently using the least amount of effort and energy possible. While this is great for day-to-day movements, efficient motions are not necessarily the best option for muscle growth. So, when you curl, your body's natural tendency is to engage the shoulders and forearms in addition to your biceps to facilitate the movement. However, this efficient, whole-arm movement reduces the work and potential gains your biceps receive from the exercise. Being inefficient, taking the shoulders and wrists out of the motion as much as possible, locks the biceps into the movement through strict form and encourages more muscle involvement—and growth.

15. **Electrical muscle stimulation (EMS)** – Stimulating your muscles with electrical impulses can shock them into growth. Some muscles respond more effectively than others to EMS training. In

the case of biceps, using EMS stimulation during your exercise routine (i.e., in conjunction with weights and intense exertion) can not only offer a novel way to train but can speed results. In this instance, EMS acts like adding additional weight and intensity to your bicep routine without the risks of additional weight (e.g., muscle tears, tendon damage, joint pain, etc.). Consider EMS another option to push yourself in new and growth-inducing ways.

16. **Blood flow restriction** – Consider wrapping your arms to restrict the blood flow to your muscle, and to increase exercise intensity and difficulty.

17. **Combinations** – Any of these variations can be combined to add variety and increase effectiveness to your bicep exercises.

18. **Be original** – Think of your own variations to add to the list.

Variety is not only the spice of life; it is also a key component of bicep growth. Use these variations and others to keep your routines fresh and your biceps growing!

Remember, this is a book about bicep-building. So, although you often need to push your limits to get your biceps to grow, you also need to be able to use them. Exercise intelligently and listen to your body to avoid injury. If you push yourself too hard, to the point of injury or inability to work out regularly, you won't be able to work those biceps and your goals will suffer.

GRIP THOSE BICEP GAINS

Something as simple as your grip can play a significant role in how effective your bicep workouts are, how targeted your exercises will be, and how much your biceps grow.

"How does this work?" you might ask.

By changing your grip, you can add additional emphasis to which parts of your arm are working and, more importantly, how hard your muscles are working as you exercise.

By changing your grip, not only can you isolate the biceps, but you can make your exercises more inefficient—that's right inefficient—to challenge your muscles and make them grow. Adding this targeted inefficiency to your exercises—and not just your bicep exercises—will make your muscles work harder, forcing them to compensate, and make them grow.

Note this focused approach to help with targeted muscles grow is different than emphasizing broad strength development where you may recruit multiple muscles and muscle groups for maximal exertion. For example, you will be able to curl more weight if you engage your forearms. You'll be able to lift even more weight if you use your torso and hips to help lift it. However, for muscle growth, there are times we may want to take as much of that assistance out of the exercise as possible, such as when focusing on a single muscle or group of related muscles, such as the biceps.

This is where good form comes into play in your exercises, such as bicep curls. Additional adjustments in the exercise, such as changing your grip, can further aid in this isolation process by making the exercise harder, more targeted, and less efficient.

Here's how to Grab Those Gains:

1. When you grip the bar, handle, or rope of your equipment, allow your wrists to rotate slightly backward. You will move your knuckles away from your body so that your forearm engagement is reduced and your biceps fully activated during exertion.

2. You will need to find an angle that does not cause undue stress on your wrists, elbows, or tendons. A slight backward tilt with a good grip is optimal. To do this, grasp the bar, handle, or rope deeply in the palm of your hand. This angle will not only ensure that your wrists and elbows are safe but it will also maximize the amount of elbow flexion generated from bicep activity.

3. You will know that you have the right grip or angle when the weight rests directly on the heel of your palm right above your wrist, and through your wrist joint and down into your forearms. When you lift the weight to the top of the exercise, you will not see the knuckles at the base of your fingers because your wrist is not curling forward—you will only see the knuckles of your fingers.

4. This grip approach is most effective when you use an appropriate weight with good form. Remember, strength requires multiple muscle groups. Hypertrophy—muscle growth —is aided by isolation. If you're lifting too heavy, your form will degrade, and you will recruit multiple muscle groups outside your biceps. Lifting lighter—but still enough to feel the exertion and work hard—will ensure that you reduce wrist, forearm, and shoulder engagement to maximize muscle gains.
Simultaneously, keeping your shoulders stable, your wrists

slightly bent, and your grip firm, will effectively isolate your biceps and fully engage your muscles.

5. Although this flexed wrist with solid grip technique is one exceedingly effective way to hold while exercising, there are others that you can use to emphasize exercises in different ways (e.g., rotating your pinkie in or out while lifting, squeezing the handle as you curl, adjusting your wrist angle, and more). Experiment and find out what works for you but always be safe!

A good way to practice this grip optimization technique is to incorporate the principles and form of Waiter's Curls into other bicep exercises.

As you know, in Waiter's Curls, the wrists flex throughout the curl while the top of the weight, barbell, or plate remains parallel to the floor through the entire range of motion. This wrist flexion focuses the majority of the exertion in the biceps and mirrors the bent back wrist approach you need to target your biceps.

Couple this wrist bend with a solid deep grip throughout your range of motion to keep you safe—holding the weight deeply in your palms and not with your fingertips—and you're going to hit those biceps like never before!

There may not be any spice in your bicep routines but variety in your grip will certainly add life to your arms!

A WORD (OR A FEW) ON SETS AND REPS

As you exercise, a common question that comes up is how many sets and repetitions should I perform for a given exercise?

The answer depends on many factors including your goals (e.g., muscle hypertrophy, endurance, definition, etc.), fitness level, age, muscular response to stress, overarching fitness routine, nutrition, and other factors.

However, without getting too complex, the answer can be boiled down to what works... what has worked for others and what is likely to work for you.

By exploring what works for yourself, not only do you keep an open mind and learn, but you also constantly work to overcome the plateaus—the lulls and setbacks—everyone faces while exercising. Further, by adding variations to those reps—and continually challenging your muscles—you open up whole worlds of possibilities beyond just worrying about sets and reps. Possibly, you'll also save yourself quite a bit of boredom.

In fact, one of the best ways to encourage continued muscular development is to change your sets and reps to keep your biceps challenged.

So, instead of thinking how many reps are "best", a more effective line of thinking may be to think about whether you are still challenging yourself and whether you are getting enough rest (both between sets and exercise sessions). Then, you can adjust the number of reps, sets, weights, exercise types, and variations accordingly.

So, while 3 sets of 8 to 12 reps of bicep exercises may be a great place to start—there's a reason so many fitness professionals and researchers recommend this range and there is some sound science behind it—this routine might not be what you need. Even the most optimal, science-based program won't necessarily work forever without adjustments—by you and in the program. If your gains have slowed and you're no longer seeing challenges in the gym, your muscles need new stimuli—or lack of stimuli, if you're overworking.

In bodybuilding, regardless of the body part, it's always advisable to hit a variety of rep ranges and even rest periods.

Typically, your reps will range from between 5 and 30 or until failure (whether this number is low or high depends on the weight involved, your fitness, and fatigue).

Generally, the relationship between the number of reps and amount of rest between sets is inversely proportional. However, this relationship also implies that those lower rep sets involve heavier weights that require more time to recover from doing. If you're lifting light and taking extended breaks between sets, you might be hanging out instead of exercising.

Here are a few examples of different rep ranges and sets along with associated rest periods that you can use to get started for your bicep exercises:

- 5 sets of 5 reps with about 120 seconds rest between sets (also known as a 5x5)
- 4 sets of 6 to 8 reps with around 100 seconds rest between sets
- 3 sets of 8-12 reps with between 75 to 90 seconds rest between sets
- 4 sets of 12-15 reps with 30 seconds rest between sets

The 5 x 5 scenario maximizes the mechanical tension placed on the muscles and is very useful in strength training. This approach does a great job of inducing protein synthesis and forcing neuromuscular improvements. 5x5 training is often used with more complex compound movements that engage multiple joints—think squats—for strength development. As an example, weighted underhand chin-ups would be ideal for bicep 5x5 training. However, this should not stop you from experimenting with other bicep exercises.

The 4 sets of 6 to 8 reps approach is one you might choose when lifting heavy to gain strength while also trying to gain mass.

The 4 x 12-15 approach maximizes metabolic fatigue and blood flow into the muscles to help create muscle hypertrophy—muscle growth and visible gains.

Finally, the 3 x 8-12 routine is an exercise classic right in the middle.

If your goal is size, you should work to stress all the various parts of the muscles' cells. Therefore, variety is crucial, not only to overcome adaptation but also to stress all muscle components. There are various ways to do this, such as spending a few weeks using one set and rep strategy at a time before switching to another, or mixing up your sets and reps in the same workout. As always, when the work becomes too easy, consider adding weight, intensity, variations, changing the time between sets, adjusting your exercise tempo, or adding more sets to keep the routine challenging.

Your biceps are like any other muscle or muscle group; the muscles in your biceps adapt to change, challenge, and stress. Overcoming and adapting to these challenges is, after all, what allows your muscles to grow, develop, and get strong.

So, not only adjusting your sets and reps but also finding which changes are most effective for you is a science in itself.

This process does not have to be difficult, however! Make it fun! Think of exercise like play; yes, there's some suffering but the end result—and the journey there—are totally worth it. You just need to find the right path to reach your goals. Hint... there's more than one! And don't waste any of your reps!

BE THE BICEP

Do your biceps make limp noodles look thick?

I can fix that.

All you have to do is put your mind to it.

The secret to building phenomenal biceps isn't about how much weight you can get them to move, although heavy weights can help. The secret to great biceps is *being the bicep*, feeling the bicep muscles work through the entire range of exertion, and then learning to make your muscles work effectively. Put your mind inside your muscles as you contract and relax. Put your awareness in the muscles *throughout* your exercises.

Make your muscle work with your mind *and* body.

When you put your mind into your muscles, you're not just watching; you're engaging. This attention gets you to work, not watch. And not just work, either. This attention helps you work more fully, harder than you would otherwise.

Use your awareness to enlist more muscle fibers, to stimulate the right muscles, to correct improper form, and to push harder and more completely than you would when just counting reps or holding a position for time.

Fully engaging in your exercises will not only focus your attention, it will also stimulate your muscles through greater activation, help you observe opportunities for improvement, show you ways to improve your form, give you ideas for ways to make your exercises more effective, and spur your muscles on to greater growth.

Biceps are no exception. Connect the mind with your muscles to get them to grow.

Use the following techniques to build your mind-muscle connection and encourage bicep growth... or come up with your own:

1. **Weighted Bicep Flexes** – Sit down in a chair with your feet placed flat on the ground. Let your arms hang relaxed by your sides. Now, pick up a dumbbell with each hand. Maintaining as much relaxation throughout your body as possible, curl the weight up one arm at a time. Try to use only the muscles in your biceps to lift. Concentrate on your biceps to the point where your biceps seem like the only muscles in your body. At the top of your curl, hold the contraction for 10 seconds. Tighten your muscles, flexing as hard as you can while supporting the dumbbell as you hold. Repeat, performing 3 to 4 bicep flex curls per side. The more seated bicep flexes you perform with full attention, the better your mind-muscle connection will be. Alternatively, perform the same routine while standing. For more challenge, add more weight or hold your flexed contractions for longer. Bring this same level of concentration and focus to your other bicep exercises to fully take advantage of the movement and activate those muscles.

2. **Flex** — Yes, flex! Whenever you're standing—or sitting—in one place for extended periods, contract your arms and flex. Hold this position until your biceps start shaking (i.e., perform an extended isometric bicep contraction). This isometric hold is perfect for when you're sitting or standing at your desk or counter, working at a benchtop, seated at work, waiting in a meeting, or performing any other activity that has you staying in place. Flexing in place is also a great way to boost the mind-

muscle connection with your biceps—and your gains! I do recommend trying to be subtle about this. When you're at work, you may not want to be on stage for more reasons than one.

3. **Every Day is Bicep Day** – I mean it! Every time you work out, perform one set of exercises for biceps. You can do this set on any suitable equipment using any bicep-focused exercise. Be creative and focus on building your mind-muscle connection as you work, so that working your arms—and engaging them fully —is part of your normal routine.

4. **Slow Motion Curls** – Do one bicep curl. That's it! Just one. Except you're going to do your curl as slowly as possible. Try to do one curl over 60-seconds. If 60-seconds is not long enough to fully tax you, try 90 seconds or two minutes. As your strength and mind-body connection improves, extend the length of the bicep curl. Put your mind in the muscle, focus completely, and breathe. As the pain and discomfort grow, you won't be able to do much other than focus on those burning biceps! And, this extended time under tension will become time for gains.

The mind-muscle connection is exceptionally important for muscle growth, especially with the biceps. The mind-body connection, particularly learning to use this connection effectively, is also one of the weakest links in most people's overall fitness practice. Strengthen the mind-body link and your biceps will begin to become the ideal you dream of every day.

GENERAL BICEP ROUTINES

Beastly Biceps is filled with bicep exercises and variations that you can combine to blast your biceps into the stratosphere. However, if you need some ideas on where and how to start those exercise routines, or how to connect exercises to make a program, this chapter will give you a few ideas to start and build upon.

Subsequent chapters will give routines and options that are a bit more unique.

Beginner's Bicep Program

This simple, introductory program is for people who have never lifted before. Focus on maintaining good form throughout each rep, putting your mind in the muscle, and getting comfortable with the exercises.

The program focuses on doing two bicep workouts each week with at least two days of rest between sessions. Each routine involves only one exercise. You can do this program up to three or four months, until you feel ready to advance, or when you are no longer challenged and need to make adjustments to see gains. To make the routine more challenging, add more weight, adjust your tempo, or intensify your bicep contractions. Alternatively, you can combine the two days into one to try a different routine.

Workout 1:

EZ bar curls - Perform 3 sets of 10 to 12 reps, resting two minutes between sets.

Workout 2:

Standing dumbbell curls - Perform 3 sets of 10 to 12 reps, resting two minutes between sets.

Advanced Beginner's Bicep Program

If you're more familiar with lifting, or want to start with a greater challenge, this beginner's workout is a good place to start.

As with the beginner's workout above, this program focuses on two workouts a week as you build strength and ability. You can do this program for up to three or four months, until you feel ready to advance, or when you are no longer challenged and need to make changes to see gains. To make the routine more advanced before moving on to another routine, use similar options discussed in the beginner's workout above, including adding weight, adjusting your tempo and contractions, and combining workouts into a single session.

Workout 1:

1. **Barbell curls** - Perform 2 to 3 sets of 10 to 12 reps, resting two minutes between sets.

2. **Hammer curls** - Perform 2 to 3 sets of 10 to 12 reps, resting two minutes between sets.

Workout 2:

1. **Preacher curls** - Perform 2 to 3 sets of 10 to 12 reps, resting two minutes between sets.
2. **Cable curls** - Perform 2 to 3 sets of 10 to 12 reps, resting two minutes between sets.

Intermediate Bicep Program

This intermediate routine involves a bit more volume and intensity than the beginner's workout. As with the beginner's and advanced beginner's workouts above, there are two workouts in the intermediate program.

However, instead of performing two workouts a week, you will choose one of the two intermediate workouts and alternate your workouts weekly.

You can do this program up to four to six months, until you feel ready to advance, or when you are no longer challenged and need to make modifications to see gains. As you grow stronger, increase weight, intensity, add variations, or move on to another routine.

Workout 1:

1. **Barbell curls** - Perform 3 to 4 sets of 6 to 8 reps, resting two minutes between sets.
2. **Seated dumbbell curls** - Perform 3 to 4 sets of 10 to 12 reps, resting two minutes between sets.

Workout 2:

1. **EZ bar curls** - Perform 3 to 4 sets of 10 to 12 reps, resting two minutes between sets.
2. **Concentration curls** - Perform 2 sets of 20 reps, resting two minutes between sets.

Advanced Intermediate Bicep Program

This advanced intermediate routine amps up the volume and intensity further and lays the groundwork for more advanced programs. This routine combines the exercises in earlier iterations into one muscle-building whole.

Use this program for up to four to six months, until you feel ready to advance, or when you are no longer challenged and need to make alterations to see gains. As you grow stronger, increase weight, intensity, add variations, or move on to another routine.

Workout:

1. **Barbell curls** - Perform 3 to 4 sets of 6 to 8 reps, resting two minutes between sets.
2. **Seated dumbbell curls** - Perform 3 to 4 sets of 8 to 10 reps, resting two minutes between sets.
3. **EZ bar curls** - Perform 4 to 5 sets of 8 to 10 reps, pausing 20 to 30 seconds between sets. This section is almost like one giant superset with short recovery breaks between sets.
4. **Hammer curls** – Perform 3 drop sets of 6 to 10 reps, resting two minutes between sets.
5. **Concentration curls** - Perform 2 sets of 20 reps, resting one minute between sets.

Advanced Bicep Program

This advanced routine raises the volume and intensity further and builds on the foundation laid by the previous programs.

Use this program for up to six to twelve months, until you feel ready to advance and push further, or when you are no longer challenged and need to adjust as you plateau.

As you grow stronger, increase weight, intensity, add variations, or move on to another routine.

Workout:

1. **Barbell curls** - Perform 3 to 4 sets of 6 to 8 reps, resting two minutes between sets.
2. **Seated dumbbell curls** - Perform 3 to 4 sets of 8 to 10 reps, resting two minutes between sets.
3. **Straight bar cable curls** - Perform 5 to 7 sets of 8 to 10 reps, pausing 20 to 30 seconds between sets. This section is almost like one giant superset with short recovery breaks between sets.
4. **Preacher Dumbbell curls** – Perform 2 sets 8 to 10 reps with slow, controlled negatives—the eccentric downward portion of the lift —resting two minutes between sets.
5. **Concentration curls** - Perform 3 sets of 20 reps, resting one minute between sets.

Alternating Weekly Biceps Workouts

This routine will have you doing one bicep routine one week and then switching to the other routine the following week. For each exercise, you will perform three sets of twelve reps. You can perform the routine as a circuit or complete each exercise before moving on to the next. If you perform the routine as a circuit—one exercise after the other—you may need to lighten your load if you are not taking enough rest to fully recover between sets.

Week 1:

1. **Biceps curls with dumbbells**: Use enough weight so that you can only do 12 reps with good form—no jerking or cheating.
2. **Preacher curls on an exercise ball or bench**: The instability of an exercise ball forces to you maintain control and avoid swinging. You may need a lighter weight as you get comfortable with the movement. Standard preacher curls are an alternative if you don't have an exercise ball to use.
3. **Hammer curls**: As you curl, rotate your palms inward to also activate your forearm muscles.
4. **Reverse curls**: Curl with your knuckles facing up to finish your routine. The combination of standard curls, hammer curls, and reverse curls will hit all your bicep heads while also working the forearms.

Week 2:

1. **Barbell curls**: Go for it! Most people can lift more with a bar, so start your routine strong.
2. **Concentration curls**: Brace yourself to fully isolate each arm and focus on those biceps as you curl.
3. **Incline curls on an exercise ball or bench**: Working at an angle, you will really feel the pull of the weights as you curl. Use that to keep your attention and work focused on the biceps.
4. **Resistance band curls**: Curls with resistance bands are not easy... if you're using enough resistance. The instability of the bands will force you to maintain focus and fully engage your muscles through the lift. Additionally, bands provide progressive

resistance—they get heavier with greater extension—so be ready to work!

Perform this routine for eight to twelve weeks for best results. Then switch this program with another routine to keep challenging yourself.

You can always come back to this routine after going to another.

Bicep Superset Routine

This routine consists of six total exercises broken down into three supersets of two similar movements. As always, you will want to maintain good form, keep your mind in the muscle, go through a full range of motion, and squeeze your biceps fully. Also be sure to follow the sets, reps, tempo, and rest periods outlined for each exercise.

Complete all sets of each superset before moving to the next superset—for variation, particularly after you have done this routine regularly for at least six weeks, you can switch to performing each exercise sequentially and add in variations.

Superset 1 – Dumbbell curls followed immediately by hammer curls.

Bicep curls – Perform 3 set of 12 reps using a 2-1-1-1 tempo with no rest after finishing (go immediately to the hammer curls). To do your bicep curls, lie on an incline bench with a weight in held each hand and your palms facing forward. Curl the dumbbells up, hold at the top, then lower the weights back down with complete control.

Hammer curls – Perform 3 sets of 15 reps using a tempo of 2-1-1-1 and then rest for 60-seconds before moving on to the next exercise. With hammer curls, use a lighter set of dumbbells than in the bicep curls that make up the first part of the superset. Lying on the incline bench with your palms facing each other while holding dumbbells, curl the weights up, hold and contract at the top, and then lower the weights with control.

. . .

Superset 2 – Preacher curls followed immediately by reverse preacher curls.

Preacher curls - Perform 3 sets of 10 reps using a 2-1-1-1 tempo with no rest after finishing (go immediately to the reverse preacher curls). Sitting at a preacher bench, hold an EZ-bar with an underhand grip, and begin curling. Lift the bar up as high as you can, hold and contract, then lower the EZ-bar slowly with control until your arms are fully extended.

Reverse preacher curls - Perform 3 sets of 10 reps using a 2-1-1-1 tempo and then rest for 60-seconds before moving on to the next exercise. Using the same weight as with your preacher curls, switch your hold to a double-overhand grip. Curl the bar up, pause at the top, and then lower until your arms are fully extended.

Superset 3 – Cable bar curls followed immediately by cable hammer curls.

Cable bar curls - Perform 3 sets of 15 reps using a tempo of 2-1-1-1 with no rest after finishing (go immediately to the cable hammer curls). Curl using a straight bar attached to the lower pulley position. Maintain good form with your elbows by your sides, raise the bar up, pause at the top, and then lower the weight under control.

Cable hammer curls - Perform 3 sets of 15 reps using a tempo of 2-1-1-1 and then rest for 60-seconds before moving on to the next exercise. For the cable hammer curls, switch the straight bar to a double-handed rope and reduce the weight by a plate or two. Grip the ropes with your palms facing one another. Curl the cable up, hold and contract at the top, and then lower the weights back down with control.

You will do this routine twice a week for six weeks, adding weight once a week to keep the biceps challenged and growing. You can incorporate this superset routine into your normal workouts as well. Just drop any other bicep exercises from your sessions if you do.

Simple and Effective Progressive Overload Routine

• • •

This bicep routine involves just three exercises to get your biceps jacked: the barbell curl, the dumbbell hammer curl, and the dumbbell curl. That's it... three exercises. Each exercise, however, should be performed at close to your maximum weight for the number of prescribed repetitions. If you can do more than the number of repetitions prescribed for a given exercise, you need to add weight.

1. **Warmup** – Get ready to lift however you choose. A few sets with light weights are one good place to start.
2. **Barbell Curls** – Perform 3 sets of 4 to 6 reps.
3. **Dumbbell Hammer Curls** – Perform 3 sets of 4 to 6 reps
4. **Dumbbell Curls** – Perform 3 sets of 6 to 8 reps

Just nine sets and you're finished. But remember:

1. If you're able to get more reps than the designated rep range for a given exercise, the weight you're using is too light. Add more.
2. Conversely, if you're not able to curl the lowest number of reps designated for an exercise, the weight you're using is too heavy. Take some weight off.

This routine is as simple as it is effective if you keep pushing yourself and adding more weight as your strength grows, so that you stick to the recommended numbers of reps.

Perform this routine for eight weeks before moving on to another.

The Working to Failure Routine

. . .

With this workout, you will use strict form to start in order to maximally engage your muscles. As the workout progresses and you tire, your strength and form will suffer, and the exercise requirements will lessen allowing your muscles to remain engaged by cheating so that you will continue pushing to your limits.

Be sure to complete all of the sets in one exercise before moving on to the next.

1. **Dumbbell curls** – Perform 4 sets of 15, 12, 10, and then 8 reps with a 60-second rest between sets. Begin from a standing position while holding a dumbbell in each hand, with your palms facing your sides. Lean forward slightly as you put your weight onto your heels. Keeping your upper arms stationary, curl the weights upward while rotating your wrists outward so that your palms face upward at the top of the curl. Squeeze your biceps for a moment as you hold at the top of the curl. Lower the weights back down back by your sides as you flex your triceps at the bottom position. Gradually increase the weight with each set.

2. **Drag curls** – Perform 4 sets of 12 to 15 reps with a 60-second rest between sets. Curl as you would for a conventional dumbbell curl but remain straight and tall as you drive your elbows back and up as you lift. The head of each dumbbell should lightly touch sides of your torso throughout the curl. Try to keep your palms facing up through the entire lift.

3. **Hammer curls** – Perform 4 sets of 15 to 20 reps with a 60-second rest between sets. Perform your hammer curls as you did the conventional dumbbell curls but keep your palms facing your sides throughout.

4. **Cheat curls** – Perform 3 sets of as many reps as possible with a 60-second rest between sets. Using the heaviest dumbbells—or barbell—you can curl, begin curling as you would for a basic dumbbell curl. As you lift, use momentum from your hips to drive through the curl and get the weight all the way up... or as high as you can manage as your arms tire. Rock your torso forward and then extend your hips forward as your torso moves

back to help complete each rep. Stop at or just before complete failure.

Bicep-Focused Standalone or Paired Routine

Do you like to focus exclusively on one body part when you work out or do you like to mix and match different body parts together? If you can't decide, then the following workouts will give you options. One focuses on a standalone bicep routine while the other can be used alongside other body parts.

The standalone routine will zero in on your biceps, exhausting supporting muscle groups as you focus on larger muscle groups toward the end of the routine. The paired biceps routine goes through the same exercises and progression but with fewer sets so that you can work other body parts alongside your biceps (e.g., triceps, back, shoulders, or anything else you choose).

Bicep Standalone Workout:

1. **Hammer curls** - Perform 4 sets of 12 reps, resting 90 seconds between sets.
2. **Biceps cable curls** – Using an adjustable cable machine with the straight bar attachment, perform 3 sets of 12 reps, resting 90 seconds between sets.
3. **Dumbbell preacher curls** – Using a preacher bench—try an inflatable exercise ball if you're working out at home and don't have a sloped bench for your arms—perform 2 sets of 12 reps, resting 90 seconds between sets.
4. **Barbell biceps curl** – Using a barbell, perform 4 sets of 8 reps, resting 2 minutes between sets.
5. **Seated dumbbell bicep curl** – Seated at a bench, perform 3 sets of 10 reps, resting 90 seconds between sets.

Paired Bicep Routine:

1. **Hammer curls** - Perform 2 sets of 12 reps, resting 90 seconds between sets.
2. **Biceps cable curls** – Using an adjustable cable machine with the straight bar attachment, perform one set of 12 reps, resting 90 seconds between sets.
3. **Dumbbell preacher curls** – Using a preacher bench—try an inflatable exercise ball if you're working out at home and don't have a sloped bench for your arms—perform one set of 12 reps, resting 90 seconds between sets.
4. **Barbell biceps curl** – Using a barbell, perform 2 sets of 8 reps, resting 2 minutes between sets.
5. **Seated dumbbell bicep curl** – Seated at a bench, perform 2 sets of 10 reps, resting 90 seconds between sets.

Much of the rest of *Beastly Biceps* will focus on unique exercises, techniques, and supplemental routines you can plug into your bicep workouts—modifying the ones here or creating your own—to get even more out of your workouts... and your development.

BICEP ROUTINES OF THE HUGE AND FAMOUS

There are many people who are famous for their physiques just as there are many famous for their knowledge. There are also some people who are famous for their biceps.

Here, I'll spread a bit of these biceps legends' knowledge so that you can enjoy their phenomenal physiques.

Arnold Schwarzenegger's Barbarian Biceps[1]

Arnold is a true legend. So are his biceps. Arnold, among many other things, is famous for developing mighty peaks that could have been transplanted directly from the Austrian Alps.

Here is one of Arnold's classic bicep routines:

- **Barbell Curls** – Perform 5 sets with 6 to 8 reps per set
- **Alternating Dumbbell Curls** – Do 5 sets with 8 to 10 reps per set

- **Barbell Preacher Curls** – Perform 4 sets with 8 to 10 reps per set
- **Concentration Curls** – Do 4 sets with 10 to 12 reps per set.

Bicep Advice from Arnold himself:

"I have discussed the technique I used to help develop my peaks so many times that it doesn't feel like a secret anymore: supination, the outward twisting of the forearm while doing dumbbell curls (you can't physically achieve this motion with a standard barbell).

Supination causes the outer head of the biceps to work hard, raising a peak and slapping on an extra bulge of muscle that you could see especially well when I did a back double-biceps pose.

When doing any dumbbell curl, whether it's standing, seated, incline, or concentration curls, start with your hand in a neutral position and then rotate it as you perform the rep so that your palm faces upward. Two inches or so from the top of the curl, twist your hand farther so that your pinkie finger is higher than your thumb and forcibly tense the biceps. The pain of the contraction is very intense, but it's well worth it. Do this with every rep of every dumbbell curl you perform, and, over the long term, it should make a big difference in your arm development.

In addition to supinating, I preferred to let the dumbbell "drag" behind to get a stronger contraction of the biceps. Most people start a curl with their wrists straight, then flex their wrists toward the shoulders for better leverage as they raise the weights. That essentially eliminates gravity and nullifies the final part of the movement, where the peak contraction can really be accentuated. But when I curled the weight, I let the dumbbell roll down my hand and settle in my fingers so that my wrist was extended throughout each rep, not flat or flexed as you usually see. This made for a longer lever arm and ensured that, even at the very top of the movement, the weight wouldn't be supported by the forearm—the tension would be on my biceps and I could really squeeze at the top. All the while, of course, I was also supinating the forearm."

• • •

Lou Ferrigno's Hulking Biceps[2]

In addition to his success on the bodybuilding stage, Lou Ferrigno is known for playing the Incredible Hulk. His biceps were pretty incredible too.

Here is one of Lou's bicep routines:[3]

- **Warm-up set.**
- **Standing barbell curls** — 4 Sets, 10 Reps.
- **Incline dumbbell curls** — 4 Sets, 8 reps.
- **Preacher-bench** — 4 Sets, 8-10 Reps.
- **Concentration curls** — 2 Sets, 8-10 Reps.
- **Barbell-curl 21s** —- 2 Sets, 21 Reps.

Bicep Advice from Lou:

"I prefer to work biceps with triceps, rather than hitting them on separate days. I usually start with biceps and finish with triceps, but sometimes I superset bi's and tri's."

Dwayne "The Rock" Johnson's Rock-Hard Arms Routine[4]

If you want to turn your biceps into boulders, the Rock's arm routine is an excellent place to start. You can always smell the Rock cooking up some huge biceps.

. . .

Here is one of the Rock's arm routines:

1. **Barbell bicep curls** – Perform 7 sets of 8-12 reps, resting 45 seconds between sets.
2. **Rope pressdowns** – Using an adjustable cable machine with the rope attachment, perform 3 sets of 8-12 reps, resting 90 seconds between sets. Be sure to pull your hands away from each other at the bottom of the exercise.
3. **Cable bicep curls** – Using an adjustable cable machine with the straight bar attachment, perform 3 sets of 8-12 reps, resting 90 seconds between sets. Alternatively, use a rope attachment.
4. **Dips** – At a dip station, perform 3 sets of 8-12 reps, resting 90 seconds between sets. Add chains or weights for added difficulty.
5. **EZ bar curls** – Using an EZ bar, perform 3 sets of 8-12 reps, resting 90 seconds between sets. Alternatively, perform spider curls with the same numbers of sets and reps.
6. **Close-grip barbell bench presses** - Using barbells at a bench, perform 3 sets of 8-12 reps, resting 90 seconds between sets.
7. **Dumbbell preacher curls** - Using a pair of dumbbells at a preacher bench station, perform 4 sets of 8-12 reps with no rest before the next exercise. These dumbbell preacher curls are performed as a superset with the reverse curls below.
8. **Reverse curls** - Using a barbell, perform 4 sets of 8-12 reps, resting 45 seconds between supersets. These reverse curls are performed as a superset with the dumbbell preacher curls above.
9. **Overhead triceps extensions** – Using a dumbbell, perform 7 sets of 8-12 reps, resting 45 seconds between sets.

Training biceps with dedication has helped make the careers—and bodies —of the world's most elite bodybuilders. Even if you're not a bodybuilder, take the advice of some of the world's best bodybuilders to get your biceps to grow!

ENTER THE PAIN BOX

This workout is as simple as it is grueling. You will come to know pain and you will work through it. You will fail and you will work through it. Through your pain and failure will come success—the beastly biceps you're willing to suffer for and fail to achieve.

With the Pain Box, you will work your biceps for three minutes. That's three minutes under tension for your biceps to grow. More time under tension is great for muscle growth.

The idea of the Pain Box is to work, to get the blood flowing into your muscles, and to push not just *to* but *past* failure. Your form will decline. You will not be able to perform full repetitions. Your partial repetitions will become partial movements.

Your partial movements will become isometric holds.

Your isometric holds will become isometric drifts.

This failure is expected and is the foundation of the exercise. As long as you are working, as long as you have not let your arms relax, straighten, and fall by your sides, you are still in the 'pain box' and performing the exercise routine properly. Do not give up until your time is up! Stay in the pain box to achieve those gains.

And, when your torture has finally ended and you've gotten a blessed reprieve, your workout is done.

. . .

Here's how to enter the pain box:

1. You'll need a timer to help set your workout pace.
2. Warm up to get the blood flowing and activate your muscle. Jumping jacks, pushups, jogging in place, a few light curls, or anything else that gets you ready and engaged should work.
3. Choose a weight that will be challenging for the entire session. You can start with a weight that is about 40 to 60% of your one rep max. If that is too easy or light, you can always use a heavier weight.
4. You can use dumbbells, a curl bar, a cable, bands, or anything else you want to lift (and that will tolerate you lifting it).
5. Find a position that is comfortable and that helps reduce cheating. With a cable, you might lie down on the floor and curl with the cable between your arms. With dumbbells, you might find a chair or bench that supports your back, that you can lock into to minimize movement. Standing, you could lean against a wall to reduce rocking. Just find a comfortable position that you can't run from once you enter the pain box.
6. For one minute, perform regular controlled curls (i.e., standard basic curls straight up and down with the weights in front of you), at roughly shoulder width. Use good, slow form. Immediately switch to the next exercise after one minute.
7. For one minute, perform curls with a wide grip using good form —or the best you can give. Immediately switch to the next exercise after the second minute.
8. For one minute, perform curls with a narrow or close grip with the best form you can. Do your best to work through the fire raging in your arms.
9. While curling, *do not stop exerting for the entire work period*. Even if that means you are just holding the weight in place as it slowly drops toward the floor, do not stop exerting! If you cannot lift, hold. If you have to, you can even fling the weight up—only

after you absolutely can no longer lift it—and then resist the weight going back down. Do not relax your muscles until the time is up!

10. The point of the pain box is to never stop exerting, to stay in the pain box for the whole three-minute period.
11. Relax, stretch, and appreciate the absence of pain when done.
12. You've made it and your bicep work is done until the next session!

As always, use any variations you want once you enter the pain box. For instance, change the order of the lifts, alter your hand rotation, change your rate of lift, add weight, add holds at peak contraction, or just use the same lift for the whole three minutes...whatever will make the pain box more painful. By painful, I mean effective.

Do not cheat or quit! You're not doing this to impress anyone else.

You're entering the pain box to make yourself better.

Pushing through adversity is one surefire way to add resilience and mental fortitude. Your biceps aren't the only things that grow with the pain box.

The Pain Box is torture. That's the point. But it is also a great exercise for your biceps. And, once you step outside of the box, your gains will be clear for all to see.

HIIT THOSE BICEPS

High intensity training is generally considered to be training involving periods of exercise at or near maximal exertion followed by short periods of rest.

These rest periods generally do not provide enough time for full recovery from the intense exertion of the exercise.

Tabatas, for example, are one type of HIIT training where you go through one or more intense exercises over a four-minute period. Tabatas involve eight twenty-second exertion phases broken up by eight 10-second rest phases right after exertion. So, over four minutes, you exert yourself at or near maximum effort for 20 seconds and then take a 10-second break eight times in the four-minute Tabata set.

Tabatas and HIIT can make great bicep-building challenges. They allow you to throw short, intense bursts of exertion at your arms. You could, for example, mix up as many arm exercises as you can think of in a single HIIT session or just focus on one.

Here are a couple of bicep-specific HIIT routines.

Consider these as idea starters as you fill in your own routines.

The options here are truly limitless. If you want to broaden these programs to work the entire arm, consider adding triceps, shoulder, and forearm work into the rotations.

.   .   .

Tabata session 1:

One of our favorite HIIT sessions involves drop-set Tabatas with standing barbell curls. If you don't have access to a gym with all the various bars, weights, and cable systems, you can use bands or dumbbells at home for this routine. After warming up, for 20 seconds, perform normal single- or double-armed bicep curls with the maximum weight you can handle for 8 to 12 reps. Follow the normal Tabata protocol of 20-second exercise phases followed by 10-second rest phases for 4 minutes. When you can no longer lift your weight with good form, drop to a lower weight during the next rest cycle and keep pushing in the following exercise phases. Drop weight as you hit failure in your sets but only as needed—you're not trying to take the challenge out of the Tabata. If your biceps are not on fire after eight successive sets with minimal rest between, you're not trying hard enough, aren't using enough weight, or aren't using good form.

Tabata session 2:

Another of our favorite HIIT sessions involves Tabatas with standing barbell curls, going through a range of different curl types for each exertion phase. As with HIIT session 1, if you don't have access to a gym with all the various bars, weights, and cable systems, you can use bands or dumb-bells at home. After warming up, for 20 seconds, perform normal single- or double-armed bicep curls with the maximum weight you can handle for 8 to 12 reps. For each 20-second exercise period, choose a different exercise to hit those biceps from all angles with minimal rest. Any exercises presented in this book will do.

Examples you can use are hammer, close grip, wide grip, normal grip, concentration, preacher, and drag curls. Variation can be added in by rotating your hands in and out from the neutral palm-up position, performing single or double-armed curls, curling across your body diagonally, speeding up or slowing down reps, adding pauses within the curl movement, and more.

Note:

As you suffer through a Tabata session, because you are working so hard, you may not be able to think as clearly and effectively as normal. As a result, you may want to plan out your exercises before you get started so you're not struggling to think of what to do next when you're exhausted and in pain and have only 10 seconds to think of what to do next.

Much like the Pain Box, HIIT training pushes you to your limits in short, intense time periods. As such, you may need significant recovery time after HIIT sessions. But your biceps won't know what hit them.

PARTIALS FOR PAIN—AND GROWTH

In this routine, you are going to prime your muscles for failure. After you've primed the pump for muscle growth, you'll push through the pain and work some more to blast your muscles into oblivion. This superset starts with partial reps and then moves to full range reps after you've burnt your muscle out.

You may hate me for putting you through this routine, but your biceps will thank me...after they've recovered and you're done crying on the floor.

Here's a partial rep superset routine that primes your biceps for gains:

1. **Weight Selection and Preparation** – After warming up, choose a weight that allows you to maintain good form throughout the exercise range. You will be performing partial reps to start, so you need to choose a weight that you can hold in place with your arms at a 90-degree angle.
2. **Partial Reps** – Starting with your arms holding the weight at a 90-degree angle, perform partial reps to failure. Move the weight

up and down slightly above and below the 90-degree angle. Remember, you are not performing full reps. You are priming the muscles for growth, getting them full of blood to build a pump, and prefatiguing your muscles.

3. **Full Reps** – When your arms are on fire and you cannot perform any more partial reps, *immediately* switch to normal curls over the full movement range. Aim for a target number of repetitions (e.g., 8 to 10, 10 to 12, or 15 to 20). No matter what, perform all of your target reps. Your form will be terrible and it will get worse as you go on, but the blood will be flowing and your muscles will grow.

As you perform this routine, consider adding variety to keep the workout fresh, encourage engagement, avoid mental exhaustion, and to continue shocking those biceps. You can change your grip (e.g., palms up, down, or to the side), the weight used, the type of apparatus (e.g., dumbbell, curl bar, kettlebells, barbell, pulleys, bands, etc.), the exercise performed (e.g., standing curls, seated curls, hanging curls, etc.), the exercise tempo, and any other variation to keep those gains coming.

The Partials for Pain workout is yet another way to fully fatigue your muscles, fill your biceps with rejuvenating blood, force you to work through the pain and exhaustion of hard exercise, and shock your muscles into growth.

Remember, the path of suffering, exhaustions, and exertion leads to beastly biceps!

THE THREE-SECOND SQUARE

You've entered the Pain Box, you've HIIT those biceps, and you've done Partials for Pain. Now. Now you're going to enter the Three-Second Square to blast your biceps right out of the box.

The Three-Second Square is simple. You perform curls lifting three seconds up, holding for three seconds at the top, going down for three seconds, and holding for three seconds at the bottom. The Three-Second Square is a whole different kind of Pain Box, one you want to get in to get those biceps to grow.

Here's how to enter the Three-Second Square:

1. After warming up, choose a weight that is manageable. You're not trying to set any records here. With the Three-Second Square, you're controlling the weight, never letting your muscles relax. If the weight is too heavy, you lose control. Start with a pair of 20- to 25-pound dumbbells. If that sounds light, then you haven't tried the Three-Second Square.
2. As you lift with your palms up in a standard curl, lean forward

slightly—being seated helps here. Leaning forward helps concentrate your peak contraction to engage the bicep more fully. Raise the weight for three seconds.

3. Hold the dumbbells at peak contraction for three seconds. Maintain tension in your biceps as you hold the weight tightly.
4. Lower the weight slowly for three seconds. Lean back slightly as you lower to settle the weight into your biceps. Control the weight on the way down, maintaining tension in the muscles.
5. Hold at the bottom for three more seconds. Do not fully straighten your arms! Maintain a slight bend to keep the tension in your muscles. That's one rep. Go until failure.

The Three-Second Square keeps your biceps in an intense, high exertion box that they cannot escape. The only way out is to work and grow.

As always, as your body adapts, add intensifiers to prevent plateauing and stimulate continued growth. You can make it the Four-Second Square, the Five-Second Square, use heavier weights, adjust your hand positions, or any other variation that works. But, whatever you do, don't leave the Three-Second Square until your work is done.

DRAG YOUR BICEPS FOR GAINS

This superset takes two variations on drag curls, joins them together, and ignites your biceps on fire for pain-induced gains.

The first portion of the superset is a traditional drag curl where the weight (i.e., dumbbells, barbell, or cable) follows your torso up and down with each curl. The second portion of the superset is a modified drag curl where you perform a standard curl lifting the weight up normally, but perform a drag curl on the way down, letting the weight follow your chest and stomach on the way down with a bar, or your sides with dumbbells.

Here's how to drag curl your biceps for gains:

1. Choose a weight that allows you to work throughout the entire range of your bicep contraction for 20 reps. You're not trying out to be the World's Strongest Man. You're here to light your biceps on fire and you'll need a weight that you can handle.
2. You will be performing one giant curling superset composed of two different variations of drag curls. Your target is 20 reps with each portion of the superset. If your arms aren't on fire with your

last reps, keep going until failure and consider adding more weight, slowing down, or adding pauses/holds into the movements.

3. Perform 20 standard drag curls using good form, letting your torso be the guide for your weights as you curl upward and your elbows move back to accommodate the drag motion. Be sure to maintain contact with the weights and your body as you curl and don't let your elbows flare outward. Your elbows should be straight back and in line with your body.

4. After completing all your reps, immediately switch to a standard curl-drag curl hybrid for 20 additional reps. Keep your elbows locked in at your sides and do not rock as you curl the weight up toward your shoulders. On the way down, allow your elbows to shift backward into the drag curl motion as the weights follow your torso down to your waist. With this drag curl variation, your arms will be making a rough semicircle as you curl, going out and around on the way up and straight down while lowering.

5. These curls become more and more difficult as your muscles tire and the pain builds. Push through the discomfort and maintain the best form you can, even as it deteriorates.

As with any exercise, use your creativity to find new challenges and variations to not only keep your muscles growing and strength building but also to avoid boredom and lack of motivation. Variations you can try range from adjusting weight, changing curl types (e.g., drag on the way up and curl on the way down), altering lift tempo, accentuating the eccentric or concentric phases of the lift (i.e., the negative or extension and the positive or contraction), adding pauses at the top, bottom, or middle of the lift, changing the weight type (e.g., using dumbbells, a barbell, an EZ curl bar, cables, bands, or ropes), and others.

However you decide to perform the superset, always do your best and keep pushing!

PUSH TO FAILURE AND THEN PUSH SOME MORE

In the world of physical fitness, bodybuilding, and personal development, failure is your friend. The more you fail, the more you gain... sounds a bit like life, doesn't it?

Working with your biceps is no different.

This superset workout forces you to reach absolute failure over and over. Each set focuses on different portions of your bicep muscles, making sure your entire bicep complex has the same stimulus for growth—total failure.

Here's a triset routine that pushes you to curl to failure:

1. Choose a weight that allows you to work throughout the entire range of your bicep contraction (e.g., a weight you would lift for a set of 8 to 10 reps). If a weight is too heavy, you won't be able to lift it fully and completely engage the muscle. Again, you're not here to impress anyone. You're here to work.
2. You will be performing one giant curling superset composed of three different curl types. For each curl, lift until absolute failure.

That is to say, you will curl until you can barely lift the weight—partial reps are fine.

3. Curl to failure with:
4. Reverse grip (knuckles up) curls,
5. Close/narrow grip curls (palms up), and
6. Wide grip curls (palms up).
7. Do each move immediately after the other. You're just changing your hand positions between sets. There are no breaks until you are done with all three exercises.
8. Each move becomes progressively harder as you fatigue and the burn builds. Do not give up! Pain is your friend here. Pain leads to growth and development.

When you're done, you will have found yet another way to enter the pain box and shock your biceps into growth.

As your strength increases and you grow more comfortable with the routine, add variety to keep the moves fresh and continue forcing your muscles to grow. Use any variations you want from adjusting weight, changing curl types, altering lift tempo, accentuating the eccentric or concentric phases of the lift (i.e., the negative or extension and the positive or contraction), adding pauses at the top, bottom, or middle of the lift, and others.

CLIMB THE PYRAMID... BUT DON'T FALL OFF

Climbing the Pyramid is as simple—and effective—as it is painful. This routine follows a giant pyramid superset where you choose a starting weight, curl to failure, and then add more and more weight while reducing reps until you cannot curl any more.

Then, when you've reached your limit, you drop the weight and increase the reps, and curl until you're back where you started.

You'll ascend in weight but go down in reps, and then descend in weight but up in reps to complete the pyramid.

Your biceps will be on fire but that pain will be the fuel to more growth.

Here how to Climb the Pyramid:

1. Climbing the pyramid works best with equipment where you can quickly and easily adjust the weight you're curling between each set. If you have adjustable dumbbells at home—or no competition for dumbbells at the gym—or a pulley machine for cable curls, you're good to go.
2. After warming up, choose a starting weight that you can curl

about 20 times. When you curl, lock your elbows in place so you're only lifting with your biceps. Squeeze through the whole lift, particularly at the top. The seated cable curl works great here because you can lean back and allow your body to define the limits of the curl while remaining stationary, with your knuckles hitting your thighs at the bottom and your chest or shoulders at the top, depending on your grip.

3. After completing your first set, quickly choose the next weight up on the pulley machine or dumbbells. Perform as many good reps as you can until failure at this weight.

4. Go up to the next weight and repeat. Then repeat some more.

5. Continue performing as many good repetitions as you can until failure at each weight level. Your form will deteriorate as you push through your curls and the weights go up. When you can barely perform 3 partial reps at your max weight, drop the weight and cycle back down toward your starting weight. Perform as many reps at each weight as you can with the best form you can manage.

6. Thank—or curse—me when you're done.

Once you've Climbed the Pyramid and seen what the view from the top has to offer, add isometric holds at the top or bottom, increase your weight, increase your reps, extend the time lifting and lowering the weight, adjust your hand positions, or use any other variation to keep those gains growing.

Climbing the Pyramid will give your biceps peaks even the pharaohs of old would admire, and, like the pyramids, they will stand up to the test of time.

INCLINE THOSE GAINS

Incline Those Gains is a seated bicep superset that will use your body's position at various angles on an incline bench to hit your biceps from multiple directions and shock your muscles into growth.

You will curl until failure from one position, adjust your body's angle, and then keep curling as you shorten the angle of your lift leaning forward.

Here's how to Incline Those Gains:

1. You're going to perform three sets of curls, one right after the other. The first set will be leaning back with your arms hanging straight down for a maximum range of motion. The second set will be performed sitting straight up with your arms hanging by your sides. The third set will be performed leaning forward with your arms hanging down and your range of motion limited by your torso, to focus on the biceps' peak contraction as you curl.
2. For the first part of the superset, using an adjustable weight bench, set the angle on the incline bench backward slightly past 90 degrees so that you are leaning back when performing your

seated curls. This slight decline will force you to go through a full range of motion and help make sure the tension of the lift is kept in your biceps and not your shoulders.

3. Sitting at the adjustable bench with dumbbells, you can curl about 20 times, lean back, and let the weights hang by your sides. Perform 20 full-range incline curls with your palms facing up.

4. For the second part of the superset, immediately sit straight up and perform another 20 curls. Curl up from your waist as high as you can. As your form begins to fail, keep pushing and lift as best you can.

5. For the third portion of the superset, lean forward without resting and perform another 20 curls focusing on the pump of your bicep contraction. Keep your mind in your muscles as you lean into the curls and try to maintain good form, focusing on your bicep's peak contraction as you curl.

6. You've worked through a range of angles from long to short and can cool down and stretch, or move on to the next exercise to blast your biceps, arms, or whatever else you're working.

For an added challenge, add another set, perform the routine in reverse, incorporate isometric holds at the top or bottom of your curls, increase the range of angles you curl through, increase your weight, extend the time lifting and lowering the weight, adjust your hand positions, use another piece of equipment, or any other variation that makes you work.

Incline Those Gains works your biceps from multiple positions all in one glorious sitting. Incorporating this superset into your arm routine along with other options presented here will keep your biceps off-balance and growing from every angle.

DECLINE THOSE GAINS

You've Inclined Those Gains, now let's decline them! Decline Those Gains is a seated bicep superset that will make you think you're climbing a mountain that doesn't end. You're going to lift until failure and then, you guessed it, lift until you fail some more.

Here's how to Decline Those Gains:

1. Using an adjustable weight bench, set the decline slightly past 90 degrees so that you are leaning back when performing your seated curls. This slight decline will help make sure the tension in your arms as you lift is kept in your biceps and not your shoulders.
2. Sitting at the adjustable bench, lean slightly back and let the weights hang by your sides. Begin by performing full-range incline curls with your palms facing up. Do not let your arms fully straighten as you lower the weight back so that your biceps remain engaged throughout the exercise. A relatively light

weight is fine here—twenty to twenty-five pounds—less than you would normally curl.

3. Perform incline curls until you cannot lift any more.
4. Without stopping and while remaining seated, transition to drag curls—lifting the dumbbells up with your elbows first instead of your hands—until you can't lift any more.
5. You've reached the end of your decline and can cool down, stretch, or move on to the next exercise.

For added suffering—growth potential—add isometric holds at the top or bottom, increase your weight, extend the time lifting and lowering the weight, adjust your hand positions, combine with other exercises, or add any other variation that makes you work.

Decline Those Gains hits your biceps until they fail and then hits them some more. Just don't fall off the cliff—or bench. I want your biceps to grow, not break.

PULL AND DRAG FOR BIGGER BICEPS

Like any muscle, your biceps respond to work. This routine, much like Decline Those Gains, combines a standard dumbbell curl with a drag curl to create a super superset which will get your biceps to work—and then work them some more.

This superset is so effective because the routine not only maximizes time under tension but it also allows you to keep working your biceps through fatigue with a slightly different movement. You may hate the continued exertion but your biceps will love it!

Here's how:

1. Choose a lighter weight than you'd normally select for your dumbbell curls. Twenty to twenty-five pounds is a good place to start (or less than half what you'd normally curl when lifting heavy).
2. Perform standard curls to complete failure. Lift from your hands, keeping your shoulders and upper arms stationary. Bring the weight as high as you can while controlling the weight as you

move it up and down. Contract your biceps tightly at the top. Don't rock or cheat as you lift. The lighter weight will allow you to maintain good form and solid muscle involvement throughout.

3. Once you're completely fatigued and can no longer do standard curls, switch to drag curls using the same weights. Keeping the head of the dumbbells by your sides, lift the weights up from beside your hips, dragging the weights along your torso, and bring the dumbbells up to your armpits. Remember, you're lifting with your biceps, not your lats. Feel the weight in your arms, not your back. Squeeze your biceps on the way up and at the top of the lift. Control the weights on the way down as you lower them along your sides once more. Don't let the weight drop. Keep dragging those weights until your biceps can't lift any more.

With the double failures in this curl-and-drag superset, your biceps will enjoy twice the success—and pain—of normal curls. To keep your curl superset interesting, use other weights like a barbell, EZ bar, or cables for the lifts. If you're feeling really good, combine the pull and drag superset with other bicep routines in this book to create a bicep workout. If you're feeling great, add those other exercises as part of a bicep-destroying super-set. The pain won't be as memorable as your smoking guns.

LOCK YOUR SHOULDERS TO LOCK IN THOSE GAINS

Many bodybuilders, fitness enthusiasts, and exercise aficionados are well aware that using momentum to cheat can, if not used properly, negatively impact gains.

However, not as many are aware that not only can you cheat by rocking your hips and torso to assist with lifts, but also that your shoulders can play a role in cheating. Pushing and rotating forward from your shoulders can not only assist with lifts but also shorten your range of motion.

Similarly, curling up from the wrists, while good for forearm engagement, can interfere with bicep movements. Not only can curling up with your hands and waist initiate momentum but this curl, as with extra shoulder involvement, can shorten the range of your curl. Taken together, hands, wrists, and shoulder engagement can lessen your biceps' range of motion, exertion, and growth potential.

Use the waiter's curl to overcome momentum issues, encourage a full range of motion, and ensure only your biceps are working throughout the lift. This unique lift will focus the benefits of your exercise on the muscles you're targeting—the biceps!

Here's how:

1. Pick up a pair of dumbbells that are lighter than those you normally use for curls. Using lighter dumbbells will reinforce the good form that waiter's curls encourage, break old habits, and unlock growth potential.

2. Perform one set of waiter's curls until failure. Make sure your posture is vertical—no leaning forward to shorten the curl motion. Curl up, keeping the head of the dumbbell flat and in line with the ground—the handle will remain perpendicular to the floor. Holding your hands flat with your palms up helps here. If you're rotating your palms upward to break the plane of the ground—not keeping your palms and the dumbbell head parallel to the ground—while you curl, or if you are engaging your shoulders, you're not getting the most out of this exercise. Try to lift the weight straight up in line with your body—not in an arc in front of you.

3. Rest and perform another two sets as above until failure.

4. You can add this routine into your arm day or perform the routine on its own as part of your regular exercise regimen.

The waiter's curl will help you overcome bad curling habits that you may not be aware you have. In the immortal words of Yoda, waiter's curls will allow you to "unlearn what you have learned" to lock in good form and unleash great gains. Then your biceps will become a true Force.

CHEAT-PROOF DRAG CURLS

Cheating isn't all bad. Cheating is actually a great way to push your limits and keep pushing when you cannot go anymore.

But this is generally done at the end of a workout or exercise, when you've already worked your muscles as much as you can through a full rep range with good form. If you start your exercises cheating, well… you're cheating!

Here's how to perform cheat-proof drag curls:

1. Load a barbell with a weight you are comfortable drag curling.
2. Bring that weighted barbell over to an incline bench, adjusted so that the bench is just about vertical—almost like a chair.
3. Rest the barbell across your thighs.
4. Grab the barbell with a neutral grip about as wide as your hips.
5. Keeping your back against the incline bench, begin your drag curls.
6. As you lift, allow the bar to slide up your stomach and torso.

7. After you've reached the top of the lift, slowly lower the weight down to your thighs.
8. Repeat the locked-in drag curls.

The beauty of these seated drag curls is that they are almost impossible to perform while cheating. Pulling back on the bar to drag the weight up your torso locks your upper body in place against the bench to prevent rocking and reduce momentum. This also ensures strict form. Keeping your back locked against the bench while seated forces your hips to stay stationary which also prevents cheating from the momentum and swinging of the weight. Having the lower rep range delimited by your thighs also reduces the amount of swinging you can do at the bottom of the curl... which, you guessed it, further reduces cheating.

Believe me, with these anti-cheat drag curls, not only will your grade school teachers be proud of your work ethic and aversion to cheating but also, your biceps will stand out proudly.

Cheaters certainly can prosper when cheating is done intelligently... at the right time and with the right intent. Otherwise, cheating can limit your growth... physically and psychologically.

ALL THE WEIGHTS DROP SET

There are so many different ways to work out your muscles that finding creative ways to exercise can be one of the most enjoyable parts of staying fit. Creating variations is not only fun but these new angles and movements challenge your body in novel ways that force adaptation and development.

And they can be fun, really fun.

Like the All the Weights Drop Set.

The All the Weights Drop Set uses dumbbells.

All of them.

Use this superset wisely or you might not be welcome at your own gym.

You've been warned.

Here's how to perform the All the Weights Drop Set:

1. Approach the rack of dumbbells proudly and announce your intentions—you don't have to do this step but seeing all the

weights lined up for your super superset can be quite enjoyable… like a king or queen surveying their domain. Or, you can do the polite thing and make sure no one else is going to need the weights you're about to monopolize for a few minutes. The All the Weights Drop Set is, after all, pretty obnoxious.

2. You can do this drop set with single- or double-arms in any curl type you choose. If you're concerned about time, your reputation, or being a weight hog, you may want to do double-arm dumbbell curls.

3. Choose the heaviest weight you can curl and go at it for whatever rep range you're targeting for your biceps (4 to 6, 6 to 8, 8 to 10, 10 to 12… you get the idea). Remember, lower repetitions mean higher weight and your goal is to lift all the weights!

4. Begin the curl gauntlet!

5. As soon as you complete one set of curls, immediately switch to the next lower weight set.

6. Your goal is to curl all the weights! Or curl as many as you can handle from your upper limit all the way to the feathery weights at the end that you probably never touch.

7. Depending on your strength, you might be able to touch almost every dumbbell on the rack. Then, you will have curled All the Weights!

If you're at home, you can do this superset with adjustable dumbbells, a full quiver of miscellaneous bands, or by lining up a wide assortment of random heavy objects that you can curl one after the other.

Yes, the All the Weights superset can be obnoxious but it can be fun… a challenge to put your biceps through, test your mettle, and reap the gains you work so hard to enjoy.

For variations, switch the routine around and go from light to heavy, try other equipment or movements, use cheat sets to help you lift, or any other variation that will offer a challenge.

But, no matter how silly this routine may seem, keep in mind others may need some weights too...no matter how much you may want to hog all of them.

AROUND-THE-WORLD BICEP CURLS

From the brachii to the brachialis, your biceps are made of several muscles that work in conjunction with other muscle groups. Hitting these muscles from every angle is crucial for bicep growth and development.

From the inner and outer heads of the biceps to supporting the brachialis, the Around-the-World Bicep Curls routine aims to hit all of these muscles... in one dynamic set.

Here's how to curl your way around the world.

1. Choose a dumbbell weight that you're comfortable with curling with good form, depending on your target rep range. You can use bands or cables as an effective alternative to dumbbells. As you will see, a barbell will not work for these curls.
2. A lighter weight works well here since you will be curling with your arms in various positions, especially as you get comfortable with the movement.
3. With Around-the-World Bicep Curls, you will be curling through

roughly a 180° range around your body. Each curl is performed at a different angle.

4. These curls can be done singly or with both arms simultaneously.

5. To start, keep your elbows locked by your side or sides, and begin curling with the dumbbell(s) with your arms externally rotated and your hands turned as far back as possible (i.e., your hands may be straight out from your sides or even rotated slightly behind you).

6. Adjust the angle of your curl after each rep, trying to change the angle of rotation evenly after each one. So, for example, if you are doing a set of 10 reps and moving through roughly 180°, each curl will shift about 18° from one rep to the next.

7. As you curl through the set, your hands will move from your sides to straight out in front and then beyond, to go inward across your chest to complete the full range of motion.

8. If you're up for it, go back through the same range starting from the inward angle and back out in the same set or wait until the next set.

9. To add additional variation to the curl range, change the supination and pronation of your wrists as you curl, to further accentuate the full range of exercise movements and build that burn through your entire bicep.

10. When done, both arms will have described roughly two halves of a circle around your body.

Around-the-World Bicep Curls are one of many potential variations on a basic curl routine. Instead of doing sets of curls separately inward, neutral, and outward, this approach combines them all in one set.

This superset might not be quite as enjoyable as traveling around the world but the globes you develop will be almost as nice.

PARTIAL REPS FOR FULL GAINS

The 'partial reps for full gains' program is built around a classic bicep routine called Bicep 21s. In this routine, you'll break down the bicep curl into three concentrated sections to hit all the muscles in the biceps. Dividing the curl down into its component parts allows you to curl longer, increasing time under tension which will increase metabolic stress and push those gains.

Here's how to perform Bicep 21s:

1. Standing in place holding two dumbbells, perform seven curls through the bottom half of the curl—from your thigh to perpendicular to the ground, up to your waist parallel to the ground.
2. Without stopping or relaxing the weight and your arms, curl the dumbbell upward from your waist up to your shoulders, as high as you can seven times.
3. Now that you've performed the two portions of the bicep curl—the top and the bottom sections of the movement—perform

seven more curls over the whole exercise range for twenty-one curls in total.

Bicep 21s are perfect for adding variations to hit your biceps from multiple angles. In addition to the traditional Bicep 21 routine above, try these variations to increase the burn and facilitate bicep growth:

Bicep 21s with cheat curls or forward-leaning curls:

1. While standing with two dumbbells, perform seven cheat curls or forward-leaning curls. These curls will not be through an entire range of motion.
2. Perform seven wrist rotations from an isometric hold with your arms held at a ninety-degree angle—palms facing up, rotating to palms facing down to cover wrist pronation and supination.
3. Perform seven full-range curls.

Bicep 21s with a mid-range focus:

1. While standing holding two dumbbells, perform seven curls around the mid-range of the curl—roughly forty-five degrees up and down around the middle of the curl, starting from holding your arms out at a ninety-degree angle.
2. Perform seven wrist rotations from an isometric hold with your arms held at a ninety-degree angle—palms facing up, rotating to palms facing down to cover wrist pronation and supination.
3. Perform seven full-range curls.

Add more variations by changing curl types and focus to continually shock those muscles, overcome adaptation, and prevent one of the biggest hindrances to physical development... boredom.

Bicep 21s are a fantastic way to help your biceps reach another critical number... a perfect 10. Use Bicep 21s to blast those guns into the stratosphere and encourage peak growth to take off.

BLOOD FLOW RESTRICTION TO RELEASE BICEP GROWTH

This book is full of exercises and ideas to help you get a skin-splitting amount of blood flowing to your biceps. Choices to torture your arms and get those biceps to grow include high-volume training, explosive training, heavy training, drop sets, reverse drop sets, supersets, partial sets, plyometrics, along with many others. But one of the most effective ways to influence your muscles' pump is through blood flow restriction (BFR) or occlusion training.

Elastic wraps offer a simple, easily accessible means to use BFR training on the biceps. Simply apply the wraps just below the shoulder (right above where the bicep muscle meets the shoulder). Adjust the wraps to desired tension. Experiment with the tension until the tightness feels most comfortable to you, especially if you have never used wraps before.

Wrapping your arms makes your sets more challenging. If you wrap your biceps too tightly, you'll never complete a full set—you have been warned!

You can use any exercise or machine to train with your arms wrapped... be creative as you try different exercises. If you're truly working, be prepared to test your physical and mental limits when you exercise your biceps using BFR.

When working your biceps with BFR, aim for three sets of 10 to 15 repetitions with 30-second rest breaks in between each set. The intensity of the burn you'll get with BFR bicep training will challenge your resolve. In order to help with recovery and bicep development, be sure to stretch in between sets and after—massage, heat, cold, and electrical muscle stimulation are other valuable recovery options.

Here's a basic overview of how BFR training works:

1. Do 10 to 15 full-range reps,
2. Relax and rest/stretch for 30 seconds,
3. Perform another set of 10 to 15 reps,
4. Rest/stretch another 30 seconds,
5. Finish with a final set of 10 to 15 reps, and
6. Then remove the wraps.

Work up to three rounds of these bicep killers.

When doing BFR training, be sure not to forget the second key to bicep hypertrophy—stretching. A good 30-second stretch of each bicep at the end of each set of BFR is both painful and vital.

Since you're performing standard bicep exercises with your arms wrapped, consider any variation presented in this book to increase the intensity of your exercise or shift the emphasis as you train with BFR (e.g., rep timing and cadence, adjusting contractions, adding pauses, increasing weight amount, changing the number of reps, boosting rep explosivity, altering wrap tightness, etc.). If you're lifting heavier weights, consider dropping the number of reps as well.

Your biceps will thank me when you're done... once the pain subsides.

MORE BICEP ROUTINES AND TECHNIQUES

I hope *Beastly Biceps* has your brain bursting with ideas to boost your biceps. I also hope that *Beastly Biceps* has inspired you to become just as stubborn as your biceps and willing to do everything you possibly can to get them to grow without giving up. Ever. Additionally, I hope that the programs and variations in *Beastly Biceps* have given you enough information to begin exploring new bicep-blasting routines of your own.

However, in case you need more, here are a few bonus bicep-destroying programs to keep you pushing (and bicep curling) to your ultimate goals—beastly biceps.

The Two-Minute Bicep Curl

This bicep routine is as much a challenge as it is a way to get your biceps to grow.

This routine requires you to focus on a goal and go get it. As you get stronger, you'll eventually be able to add more weight, increase your time, and find other ways to intensify the routine.

. . .

Here's how:

1. Choose a weight about 50 to 75% lighter than you would generally use for a set of 10 to 15 reps.
2. You are going to perform one curl as slowly as you can. Choose whichever type of bicep exercise you want. Make it fun! Surprise yourself!
3. Important: You are controlling the weight on the way up and down (not swinging or dropping it). Actively resist the weight pushing down into the biceps as you lower (feel the weight in your biceps as you move).
4. Time yourself going up and going down. Aim for a 30-second contraction and a 30-second extension to start. Work your way to a minute up and a minute down, and then go beyond!
5. Perform three total sets of slow, extended bicep raises.
6. Wonder if you'll ever be able to lift your arms again. Just kidding… Swinging your arms and stretching will help the soreness and stiffness go away. And the pain and development you earn will remind you why you're putting yourself through this torture.
7. For variations, consider adding contractions at the top of your curl, adding additional weight to your lift, doing a different curl type, adjusting your hand position, or increasing the length of your curl.

Bicep Brachialis Burster

As an alternative to standard curls, and a way to use a pulley machine unlike almost anyone else in the gym, consider doing reverse-grip curls on a pulley machine to really light up your brachialis… and score cool points with other gym goers.

· · ·

Here's how:

Claim your spot by the pulley machine (short sleeves to show off your gains are optional). With your feet braced for stability and your elbow held locked by your side to isolate the biceps, use one hand to curl the cable upward. Keep your knuckles facing up as you curl to really hit your brachialis.

For added emphasis, bring your knuckles up, lifting at the wrist as you curl to further hit the brachialis. You can do this either by bringing your knuckles up slowly as you curl upward in tandem with the lift or after you have finished the curl at the top of the lift. Either way—bringing your knuckles up as you curl or after you've reached peak contraction—your brachialis will burn as you emphasize the muscle.

Use whichever technique works better for you, offers the most challenge, feels the most natural, or change the technique up for variety.

For variations in the exercise, increase reps, weight, lift with two hands instead of one (i.e., using a handle or rope on the pulley), use a dumbbell or barbell instead of a pulley, reduce the rest time between sets, add isometric holds and peak contractions, and any other technique you can think of to blast those brachs!

Bicep Scorchers

If you like to work your biceps at the end of your workout but your arms are so burned out that you can barely move, then this timed seated bicep-raise workout is for you.

Here's how:

1. Standing or seated, perform as many curls as you can in a full

minute. You are not counting reps. You are pushing yourself hard for a full minute.

2. Use good form and a controlled eccentric (negative downward movement).
3. Do not stop exercising for the entire minute.
4. Do at least two sets, focusing on getting in the maximum amount of work in each minute.
5. Get a fire extinguisher ready to put out your biceps. Or stretch. We recommend stretching.
6. Add more weight, change the angles of your feet, or increase the exercise duration (which will increase the number of reps performed) to intensify the set.

Anatomically-Angled Chin-ups

To really hit your biceps and activate their growth consider chin-ups… but not just any chin-ups, rather chin-ups that are in proper alignment for your bicep anatomy.

Here's how:

Address the chin-up bar. Make sure the bar is secure if it is not fastened in place. Place your hands slightly wider than your shoulders. This will allow your arms to mimic the natural angle at which your arms rest beside your torso when carrying objects with your elbows at your side.

As you begin to put your weight on your arms, keep your elbows inside your hands to maintain this anatomical carrying angle. To further emphasize the biceps, as you grip the bar, allow your wrists to rotate slightly backward, (i.e., moving your knuckles away from you and the heel of your palms up) so that your forearm engagement is reduced and your biceps are fully activated during exertion.

When you begin to lift up, mirroring the curling motion of a bicep curl, do not curl yourself completely over the bar with your chin close to your knuckles. Instead, raise your chin higher than the bar but keep a distance away from the bar and your knuckles. Together with proper hand and wrist placement, this will maintain the tension of the exercise in the biceps to keep them working hard as you lift.

Further, instead of pulling straight up and down when you do your chin-ups, move your body slightly away from the bar as you lower. This will help your chin-up follow the natural curving or arching motion of a bicep curl.

Chin-ups performed with proper hand and wrist placement, proper lifting form and angle, will target your biceps in a way different from conventional curls, keeping tension on the muscles throughout the lift, and overloading your biceps to help overcome your growth limitations.

For variations, consider adding weight, adjusting your lifting speed or tempo, adding pauses, changing hand and wrist position, increasing reps, and any other creative solution you can devise to bring the exercise effort into your biceps.

The Challenge

This is a simple exercise intended to push your limits. You can work this routine into other programs or perform it alone.

The Challenge is simple: perform as many biceps raises as you can with each arm. Use good form, controlling the motion without bouncing, making sure to pause at the top and bottom of each rep. When you can't perform any more full repetitions, continue with partial reps (i.e., perform partial contractions as high as you can curl or lift upward). When you've finished with one arm, switch to the other. Set a goal in mind and go for it!

Once you've hit that goal, go for more. As usual, consider intensifying the routine and throwing off your body's adaptations by increasing reps, slowing down reps, holding your stretches and contractions for longer at the bottom and top of your reps, adding weight, adding bands or chains, and any other variation that pushes you.

As an alternative, perform the Challenge with both arms simultaneously instead of one arm at a time.

Recover - Actively and Passively

Some of the routines in *Beastly Biceps* are grueling. Some approaches outlined do not give you off-days like you may be accustomed to while training. Even with traditional training, rest and recovery, along with proper nutrition, are critical to development. Rest and recovery do not have to be passive. In fact, engaging in your recovery will not only help you return to form quicker, they will also help improve your gains as you exercise.

There are a few techniques and approaches that can provide positive recovery and preventative benefits, such as:

1. Stretching (both dynamic and static).
2. Pressure, trigger point, and percussive self-massage.
3. Assisted massage (e.g., deep tissue, sports massage, shiatsu massage, lymphatic massage, reflexology, etc.).
4. Active relaxation including hot and cold baths or yoga.
5. Other relaxation, meditation, and visualization techniques.

As with the other approaches presented in *Beastly Biceps,* the important thing with these routines is to explore, experiment, and ultimately find what works for you. Once you've found what works, keep pushing to learn and do more.

Good luck and may the gains be with you!

STRETCHING

Stretching?

Yes, stretching!

Stretching your biceps, or any muscle for that matter, is a key to locking in those gains. When you stretch, not only do you get your blood flowing to help your muscles heal and grow, but also you ensure that you'll be able to use them over a full range of motion, and, most importantly, you'll be able to make the most of those gains throughout the rest of your life.

Here are a few nice biceps stretches to get you prepared to blast those biceps, build your bazookas, help your arms recover, and get you living the best life possible—showing off those guns!

1. **Modified child's pose** – For all you yogis out there, this stretch is for you. For all of you non-yogis, this stretch is for you too…and your biceps. Sit down on the floor on your shins with your feet tucked under your buttocks. Lean forward at the waist and let your torso rest on your thighs. Reach both arms forward to full length and press your palms on the floor. Extend both arms out and slightly to the side—forty-five degrees or less—keeping your palms on the floor. Push your torso downward into your

chest to create tension and extension of your muscles. You should feel this stretch in your chest. To hit the biceps, rotate your hands inward until the inside knuckle and index fingers are touching the floor—like a knife hand for you martial artists. Push your arms downward toward the floor. This will extend your arm and put tension in your bicep. You can also rotate your shoulders slightly to further emphasize the stretch.

2. **Wall stretch** – Find a wall, doorframe, piece of gym equipment, or another vertical object. Straighten your arm and rest your hand on the wall, frame, or random vertical point of resistance. Straighten your hand and rotate it until you feel tension in the bicep. Sit with that tension and let those biceps stretch. The wall stretch is performed very much like the modified child's pose stretch, except using the wall. You can do this stretch with one arm at a time or both.

3. **Ropes and bands** – With suspended ropes or elastic bands, using one arm at a time or both simultaneously, straighten your arms under tension from the rope or band and slowly rotate your extended arm until you feel a stretch in the bicep. Once you feel that stretch, hold. Allow your weight and the tension of the rope or band to accentuate the stretch. For stability, make sure the rope or band is anchored well around an object or yourself.

4. **Weighted stretch** – Using a light weight—we're not lifting, we're stretching—lean back on a bench as if you're going to do chest flies. Holding the weight and keeping your arms straight, let your arms slowly lower toward the ground. Adjust your hand position and arm angle until you feel a stretch in your biceps.

5. **Gymnast's stretch** – Sit with your back against a chair, the couch, or a bench at the gym. Place both arms about forty-five degrees behind you, resting your hands on the seat of the chair, bench, or couch. Straighten your arms, rotate your hands inward until the sides of your index fingers are on the flat surface, and lean forward until your biceps are tight and the stretch carries through your bicep. Alternatively, place the ridge of your hand on the flat surface and scoot your bottom forward until your biceps feel the stretch. Either way, your biceps will stretch!

Almost any stretch that works for your chest can be changed into a bicep stretch with a little modification of your hand and shoulder position. All you have to do is move your body slightly until you feel the stretch in the muscle.

Play with angles to find the best stretches for you.

Now that you've worked those muscles out, go stretch, recover, and get some rest. You'll be well on your way to putting on a gun show when you're done.

WHAT'S NEXT?

What's next?

The honest answer to that question is up to you. Just as you determine how hard you work and how much success you have in life, you will also determine how much your arms grow and how well they are maintained.

Personally, I exercise my arms once to twice a week through a dedicated routine—not including other days where they're worked as a secondary muscle group. This is the level of commitment required for me to see results. Since I started working with this level of dedication, my arms have grown.

Since I am a hard gainer and don't maintain muscle mass easily, I know that if I stop exercising hard, varying my routines, and challenging myself, I will not see additional growth. I also know that if I do not work to maintain what I have gained, this progress will gradually disappear. With any luck, your road is easier than mine (hopefully much easier). But, whatever your journey, *Beastly Biceps* will get you there.

So, the choice is yours. I believe *Beastly Biceps* offers you the tools needed to help you achieve the arms of your dreams, and I hope the ideas presented have inspired you to push and strive for your goals.

Remember, your arms, like your life, are what you make of them.

I want you to keep pushing, to never stop exploring, and to continually develop.

Then, your arms won't be the only things that are beastly.

Here's to being a beast!

—Rhys Larson

CITATIONS

Here are the sources for the quotes used in *Beastly Biceps*:

1. "The Complete Arnold: Biceps." *Muscle & Fitness*, 9 June 2017, www.muscleandfitness.com/flexonline/training/complete-arnold-biceps/.
2. "Lou Ferrigno's Mass Class." *Muscle & Fitness*, 29 December 2015, www.muscleandfitness.com/flexonline/training/lou-ferrignos-mass-class/.
3. "Hulking Biceps: Lou Ferrigno Arm Workout," *Simply Shredded*, 2011, https://simplyshredded.com/hulking-biceps-lou-ferrigno-arm-workout.html
4. "Train Like the Rock: Dwayne Johnson's Arms Routine" *Muscle & Fitness*, https://www.muscleandfitness.com/routine/workouts/train-rock-dwayne-johnsons-arm-routine/.

GLORIOUS GLUTES

THE ESSENTIAL GUIDE TO BUTTOCKS GROWTH, BACKSIDE DEVELOPMENT, AND BUILDING A BETTER BOOTY

RHYS LARSON

PREFACE

A few words of caution and encouragement.

This book is about helping you reach your potential (and getting your glutes to grow). Although pushing our limits helps us—and our booty—develop and improve, we should exercise thoughtfully and with common sense.

As you work to build your backside, don't take unnecessary risks or push yourself too hard, especially not to the point of injury.

Please consult a physician before embarking on any exercise program, especially if you have any questions or concerns about your body, your health, or your exercise limitations.

I want you exercising healthily.

It's the only way to sculpt your glorious glutes.

—Rhys Larson

GLORIOUS GLUTES

Not everyone is born with the firm, round, sculpted glutes of their dreams. Whether you want a backside that is firm, round, muscular, lifted, shredded, or strong, *Glorious Glutes* can help make your dreams a reality.

For those who want to banish their sagging booty to the distant past, *Glorious Glutes* will help turn your gravity-challenged backside into sculpted perfection.

For those who want to be fit, bring variety to their exercise routines, add leg and glute development, or maintain what they have already worked so hard to attain, *Glorious Glutes* is for you too.

Glorious Glutes offers a broad range of tools, exercises, insights, and ideas to help shape and sculpt your body, particularly your glutes.

So, if you're a hard gainer who has tried everything—or think you have —to build your butt, *Glorious Glutes* will give you many novel ways to push your limits and help your gluteal muscles grow. If you're looking to sculpt and tone your bum, *Glorious Glutes* will provide you with a host of options to achieve the look you're after.

Or, if you're already jacked and looking to add a bit of variety and new options to your leg routines, *Glorious Glutes* will give you innovative ideas and programs to torture yourself both at home and in the gym.

Whether you're a fitness beginner looking for help, a seasoned body-builder or fitness professional looking for that little edge, someone who wants to get in shape, or an exercise enthusiast looking for new approaches and concepts, *Glorious Glutes* will help you improve your buttocks.

Everyone deserves a pair of glorious glutes!

HOW THIS BOOK WORKS

Glorious Glutes is built around the goal of giving you the tools and knowledge needed to get your glutes to develop and grow.

To do this, *Glorious Glutes* is broken into sections that will provide you with numerous suggestions, background information, and a wide range of exercises and routines to try. The information ranges from basic exercises you may already know to crazy ideas you've never heard of, much less tried. These routines can be performed on their own or mixed in with other exercise programs to give you the best results possible. Added into your leg days, the exercises in *Glorious Glutes* will help more than just your glutes be glorious.

Beyond basic exercises and routines, *Glorious Glutes* also offers numerous techniques and variations for each exercise to maximize development potential, novelty, and training effectiveness, as well as offering all the vital background information on how glutes work. I also include some basic anatomy to help you understand how to best to put the maximus in your gluteus.

Finally—and this is a fundamental motivation for writing this book—by bringing all these ideas and approaches together in one place, I hope *Glorious Glutes* will inspire you to experiment, explore, and learn what approaches work best for you and your overall health and fitness as you embark upon a lifelong journey toward positive living.

By learning what exercises and variations are most effective for you, I hope you will share your hard-earned knowledge and experience to help others boost their bum game and, more importantly, reach all their individual fitness goals.

Whatever buttocks targets you choose—whether it's a muscular butt or a sleek, well-proportioned booty—*Glorious Glutes* is here to make your goals possible.

BECOMING GLUTES-DEDICATED

Training any lagging body part is not easy. If your buttocks are not where you would like them to be or if they are stubbornly refusing to respond to your efforts, this frustration can lead to discouragement and interfere with your desire to reach your goals.

Although I cannot reach your goals for you, I *can* give you the tools to help you reach them. In turn, you must provide the motivation, the dedication, and the effort to bring those dreams to life. *Glorious Glutes* is also here to help ignite that spark.

Getting that fire to burn, to help you push through obstacles or disappointments and achieve the backside of your dreams will take much work, however.

Yes, *lots* of work.

This process is not simple or quick.

But you can do it.

Glorious Glutes will give you all the tools to help your glutes grow, allowing you to overcome your deficiencies and stimulate improvements. But your dedication must fuel you to reach those goals. This is the part I cannot do for you.

You *must* be committed and put forth the necessary effort in spite of any setbacks or disappointments. You *must* generate your own enthusiasm and workout regime.

Simply going through the motions as you exercise, or breezing through workouts just to get them done, will not get you where you want to be.

Your butt looks the way it does for a reason. It reflects the amount and type of effort you have put into it. So, if you haven't put in any work, or you haven't worked hard or effectively, then you haven't even scratched the surface of your booty's growth potential.

Your job, your goal, is to counter your glutes' resistance to growth and development.

No amount of knowledge or range of exercises will do anything for you if you don't make your efforts and understanding count.

Glorious Glutes will get you started on your way to the buttocks of your dreams, but *you* are the one who has to get there… one rep at a time.

I ask you to train diligently, to persevere, and to embody your end goals with each and every rep. Push to reach your dreams because no one else will—or can—do it for you.

And then you, too, will have glorious glutes.

GLUTES ANATOMY

If you want to build glorious glutes (or build up your buttocks at all), you need to understand your muscle anatomy. This way, you'll know precisely what muscles to target, recognize how to isolate them, and understand how to work toward your glute goals.

This is not to say that you won't be able to build your backside if you don't know your anatomy—because you can and you will—but rather, this means that you can help your booty grow and develop more effectively and efficiently if you do.

Trial and error works, but this approach can also be trialing, with lots of errors!

Trial with fewer errors is better.

Understanding so you can perform the *most effective* trials works best.

I want to help you avoid those inefficient trials, prevent those errors, and avoid the pitfalls that will interfere with achieving your goals.

Your buttocks are made up of many muscles, but the largest and most noticeable of them are the gluteus maximus, medius, and minimus.

The gluteus maximus is the largest single muscle belly in the human body. The gluteus maximus has a wide origin—the immobile, fixed point of muscular attachment— from the side of your tailbone up to your iliac bone (i.e., pelvis bone), and inserts—the mobile point or side of muscular attachment—into the iliotibial band on the outside of your thigh, as well as on the back of your femur (i.e., thigh bone). The gluteus maximus is the largest and outermost glute muscle, your primary hip extensor, and is the most noticeable of the gluteal muscles.

The gluteus medius is about half the size of the gluteus maximus and is mostly located beneath it. The gluteus medius originates from your iliac bone and inserts on the side of the head of the femur. The gluteus medius stabilizes your pelvis, but can also extend, abduct, and rotate your hip.

The gluteus minimus is the smallest of your three main gluteal muscles and is located underneath the gluteus medius. It originates from your iliac bone and inserts on the front of the head of your femur. The gluteus minimus aids the gluteus medius in stabilizing the pelvis while balancing on one leg. The gluteus minimus can also abduct and internally rotate your hip.

Although these are the three primary gluteal muscles, there are several more. The remaining muscles on the back of your hip are small—the size of your gluteus minimus or smaller—and deeply located. These muscles include the piriformis, quadratus femoris, obturator internus and externus, and the inferior gemellus. While they are important, these minor muscles do not contribute significantly to your glutes' total muscle mass and appearance. These muscles are also generally trained by the exercises that work your larger glute muscles.

If you want to build your glutes, now you know where to start!

ALL BOOTY, ALL THE TIME

There are well over one hundred booty-focused, glute-building exercises in *Glorious Glutes,* and this doesn't even include the many variations you can add to each movement to effectively create new exercises from traditional ones. There are, quite literally, thousands of exercise variants possible—and even more if you get creative.

Whether you focus your exercise programs on general fitness, whole-body exercises, specific sports, or targeted body-building training, the exercises in *Glorious Glutes* can be used to help you—and your body—be better, whatever *better* means to you.

One way to help you reach your glutes goals is to sample liberally from all the exercises here. Sprinkle them generously into your workouts. Try adding one buttocks builder to every workout. Whether you work out every day or three times a week, add a booty sculptor to your routine. Get in the habit of working on and challenging your buttocks consistently to build booty awareness, engagement, and development.

· · ·

If you want to develop your glutes, give them priority. If you want to turn a weakness into a strength, devote yourself to change, work creatively and strategically toward turning your liability into an asset, and put forth the effort and dedication to see your goals through.

If glutes are your weakness, make them a priority.

It's that simple.

One way to do this is working your glutes every day.

Think of the problem of helping your butt grow and develop in terms of common workout programs and goals—normal fitness frameworks and paradigms.

People go to the gym all the time, primarily for their chest days, back days, and arm days. But how often do people go to the gym for glute days?

Even on leg days, glutes are often not a focus and or are an afterthought.

When your gym buddies are bragging about their latest workout or new routine, chances are they are not talking about their glutes or everything they did on glute day.

Sure, there are numerous articles on glute exercises and programs, but the glutes are often treated as a secondary muscle group that is automatically worked during leg workouts.

With *Glorious Glutes*, I'm here to change that.

Together, we're going to make glutes a priority.

We're going to make every day glute day!

BUTTOCKS EXERCISES OVERVIEW

You may go to the gym to get ripped, to add mass, to get in shape to be able to do what you love, to build tree-trunk legs, to develop a perfect v-taper, to sculpt boulder shoulders, to create a chiseled physique, or lose some weight.

Or you may go for an entirely different reason. However, one of the most attainable—and desirable—fitness goals for many gym-goers is well-developed glutes.

The buttocks are one of the most noticeable—and noticed—body parts on anyone. In this chapter, I'll give you an overview of the wide range of buttocks exercises to get those glutes burning and the movements required to get them growing, lifted, and sculpted.

Butts are not all about aesthetics, however. Building stronger buttocks muscles will not only improve your speed and explosiveness but will also protect your lower back and knees from injury. Plus, any good butt work-out, which can and should include some of the butt exercises below, will target the biggest muscle in your body—the gluteus maximus—so you'll maximize your burn both during and after your workout.

You'll want to be sure you're working all your butt muscles—and the rest of your posterior chain—to get the most out of your efforts. The squats, deadlifts, lunges, bridges, thrusts, lifts, and jumping exercises outlined in the next few chapters accomplish all these goals and more.

How This Works

The following five exercise chapters on squats, deadlifts, lunges, bridges and thrusts and lifts, and jumps will give you an in-depth overview of specific glute-focused exercises that you can incorporate into your fitness routines. Each chapter provides enough information for you to perform the fitness routines and programs outlined later in the book or build your own.

How you use and incorporate these exercises into your booty workouts is completely up to you. See the *Exercise Variations and Modifications* chapter for a range of options for each movement and to help customize each exercise. Try a few exercises as starters or finishers for a lower-body workout, do one set each of a few for a circuit-style workout, use the moves in the routines provided elsewhere in this book, build your own program, or simply incorporate your favorite exercises into your usual full-body workouts.

What You'll Need

While you can effectively work your glutes with just your bodyweight —we're talking about pistol squats, split-stance squats, jump squats, single leg thrusts, and kickbacks—many of the exercises outlined here utilize tools and equipment that will take your glute work to the next level. Some items that you'll want to familiarize yourself with and should consider having available for your workouts are a barbell, weight plates, a set of dumbbells (I like adjustable dumbbells for quickly changing between weights and exercises when exercising at home), a squat rack, exercise bands, a weighted vest, kettlebells, ankle weights, a stability ball, a tall step or a stable box, a glute-hamstring developer machine, and a cable machine, along with a few other pieces of equipment.

Don't be discouraged by this list, however. Most of these things are available at a gym, you don't have to have everything I've listed to work your glutes, and you can be creative to keep challenging yourself with or without equipment.

Squats, deadlifts, lunges, bridges, thrusts, lifts, and jumps are a few of the many glutes exercises you can and will see used throughout *Glorious Glutes*. There are many others available, including ones you may make up yourself. Use the exercises detailed in the following chapters in conjunction with the routines outlined in this book or add them to your own routine. Coupled with variations for each exercise, and combining the exercises in novel routines, you'll have a lifetime's worth of ways to torture your buttocks.

Whatever exercises and variations you use, and however you use them, maintain good form and keep working for those gains!

A beautiful backside will soon be your reward!

SQUATTING EXERCISES

Whether you love 'em or hate 'em, squats are one of the best butt exercises that you can do at home or the gym for strengthening and developing your backside. Experts and athletes agree that if you want to run faster, jump higher, and lift heavier, squatting low is the way to go. Squats might look easy, but prepare to work hard when you add a barbell, weights, bands, a slam ball, or raised heels to the mix. These squat variations not only add some power to your jumps and kicks, they also help improve your knee stability and range of motion.

How low can you go? Try these exercises to find out.

Back Squat (Barbell Squat)

The back or barbell squat is one of the fundamental exercises for whole-body strength and muscular development, particularly for the legs and glutes. Start with the barbell on your shoulders and lower your body straight down while controlling the weight down into a seated position. Let the weight settle in your feet as you lower while keeping your chest and back upright. Control the weight and use good form throughout the movement. Don't let the weight control you. Starting and practicing good form even when lifting light weights is critical in building a solid foundation as you progress. The deeper you go, the more you'll work. There are many variations on the classic weighted barbell squat, including the Smith machine squat, hack squat, and dumbbell squats.

Front Squat

The front squat is performed exactly like the back squat except you hold the weight in front instead of behind you as you squat up and down. Unlike a back squat, where you place the barbell across your shoulders and lats, the barbell goes across your collarbone and in front of your body. This movement will force you to recruit more muscles in your core to maintain proper form. If you don't have a barbell, dumbbells, kettlebells, or bands can be used. Holding a single weight in the front turns the front squat into a goblin squat.

Goblin Squat

A variation on the front squat, the goblin squat is a whole-body, glute-burning staple. To perform a goblin squat, stand with your legs slightly wider than shoulder-distance apart while holding a weight—kettlebells and dumbbells work great here—in front of your chest with your elbows held closely to your body. Lower into a deep squat, keeping the weight held closely to your chest while pointing your elbows toward the insides of your knees. Stand up powerfully as you extend your legs while keeping your knees soft. Lower back down into the squat and repeat.

Bulgarian Split Squat

The Bulgarian split squat is one of the best butt builders in the business. If you don't believe me, add a challenging weight and do a few sets and see how your glutes feel the next day. To do Bulgarian split squats, hold a bar on the backs of your shoulders as you would for a back squat. Dumbbells work as well if you don't have a barbell or want some variety. Rest the top of your left foot on a bench, box, chair, or other stable knee-high object behind you so that your back knee is bent about 90 degrees. Bend your hips and right knee to lower your body until your rear knee nearly touches the floor. Keep your torso upright and your back in neutral position as you work. You won't need as much weight with Bulgarian squats as in a normal back squat to really work your glutes and get those gains.

Bulgarian Squat with a Slam or Stability Ball

Want to amp up your split squat? Try balancing one leg on a slam or stability ball. If you don't have a slam or stability ball, you can rest your non-working leg on another unstable object to challenge your stability muscles. With your back foot elevated, lower your weight downward balanced between your legs. A combination of a stationary lunge and a squat, the Bulgarian squat is a true leg burner. Most of the work and effort should be in your front leg as you work. Engaging your core will help keep your foot from rolling off the ball and allow you to move with control. Consider this exercise a must-do if you want a workout that offers core strengthening and a butt lift.

Suspension Trainer Bulgarian Split Squat

Like the Bulgarian squat with the slam or stability ball, the Bulgarian squat with the suspension trainer adds instability to the already challenging Bulgarian split squat. To perform, attach the suspension trainer to a sturdy overhead support and lengthen one handle so it's at about knee height. Stand facing away from the suspension trainer and rest your left foot in the foot cradle behind you. Make sure your right foot is lunge-length in front of the trainer. Bend your hips and knees to lower your body until your rear knee nearly touches the floor. Hold on to something for support if you feel you can't balance safely. Keep your torso upright—don't bend over as you lower down and stand back up. If you think you can, and your balance and strength are up to the test, add weight for even more challenge.

Stability Ball Wall Squat

The stability ball—also called the Swiss ball, balance ball, exercise ball, yoga ball, Pezzi ball, balance ball, physio ball, Pilates ball, and more besides—has almost as many names as glute-building uses. One of the best for starting your glute-developing journey is the stability ball wall squat. To do a stability ball wall squat, place the ball against a wall and stand with your back leaning against it, holding the ball in place with your weight. Place your feet shoulder-width apart and turn your toes out about 15 degrees. Squat down as low as you can, rolling the ball down the wall as you descend before standing back up. Add weights like dumbbells or a weighted vest as your strength and comfort improve.

Dumbbell Squat to Press

The beauty of compound exercise really shines through with this squat thruster. Using power from your glutes and lower body, squat down with dumbbells held at your shoulders. Press the dumbbells up overhead in one continuous movement as you stand. This move works your shoulders as well as your glutes and can really get your heart rate up for a cardio crusher.

Landmine Squat Press

Riding the line between free weights and fixed machines, the landmine is a great way to practice proper form with the squat. For those not in the know, a landmine is basically a hinged barbell that is fixed to a pivot point on one side which enables the bar to be used for a wide variety of exercises. When using the landmine, your feet should be hip-distance apart and the weight in your heels. Holding the landmine with both hands will help keep your chest upright while squatting. As you squat, lower the landmine bar to your chest. As you stand up from the squat, extend your arms and press overhead. If you don't have access to a landmine, a barbell braced to prevent sliding backward and allow pivoting as you lift should do. The landmine can be used for many other glutecentric exercises as well including various other squats and deadlifts.

· · ·

Pistol Squats

Pistol squats are single-legged squats where you hold one leg forward while you squat down and stand back up using only one leg to perform the squat motion. As you build up to an unassisted pistol squat, you can perform your single-legged squats assisted (i.e., resting some of your weight on a support or letting your nonworking leg take some of the weight) or unassisted and with your leg held forward, going out to the side, or behind you. As you get stronger, you can even add weight to your pistol squats.

Lateral Pistol Squats on a Rower

One variation of the pistol squat is the lateral pistol squat on a rower. With lateral pistol squats on a rower, you rest your non-exercising leg on the seat of a rower (or other gliding surface such as a towel on a polished floor). As you drop your weight downward, the exerting leg remains stationary below your body while the non-exercising leg glides sideways. Aside from getting in a killer cardio workout, the rower can work your booty in surprising ways. This lateral pistol squat not only ignites your glutes, but also your inner thighs and quads. You can adjust the movement by changing which direction your leg glides as you would with the single-legged pistol squat (e.g., forward or backward in addition to the side).

The Cossack Squat

Exercise like a Cossack warrior with the Cossack squat! The Cossack squat is similar to a normal squat, only you shift your bodyweight more prominently onto one leg instead of relying on both legs to squat and lift while the other leg is held straight out. To do a Cossack squat, stand up with your feet wider than shoulder-width apart. Your toes should be pointing forward, or slightly outward, but not too far out, as you work. As you descend, shift your weight onto one foot and start squatting until your hip is below the knee. Your working leg should bend as you go down, while the other leg remains straight. Your chest should be kept upright while your hips stay down throughout the movement. Drive through your foot as you push your body back to the initial starting position using your bent leg.

Cable-Assisted Pistol Squats

Great things go great together—at least in the case of the pistol squat and the cable machine. To do cable-assisted pistol squats, attach the narrow grip handle to the top of the cable machine. Alternatively, to do an unassisted cable machine pistol squat, attach the narrow grip handle to the machine at around waist height. Position yourself a few feet out from the cable machine and pull the handle towards your chest. From a standing position, holding the handle for stability, lower into a one-legged low pistol squat. Drive back up to a standing position, pushing through your heel. Perform all repetitions on one leg before switching the other side.

Front Cable Squat

A traditional squat can be modified in numerous ways to adjust the intensity, exercise focus, and safety. The front cable squat is an excellent, controlled exercise for glute development. Start your front cable squats by attaching the straight bar handle to the bottom of the cable machine. Stand facing the cable machine while holding the handle with an underhand grip. Pull the handle up towards your chest until your hands are by your shoulders or collar bones and the bar is running across the front of your chest. Engage your core and push back and down into a squat position while holding the bar against your chest. Briefly pause at the bottom of the squat and then push back up through your heels into a standing position, squeezing your glutes at the top of the movement before lowering again.

Sumo Squats

The sumo squat is much like the traditional barbell squat, except you hold your feet wider than shoulder-width apart as you squat down and come back up. This sumo/barre-inspired bodyweight squat gives you the benefits of isometric exercise by reducing the pressure on your joints. You'll not only get your glutes in gear, but your hamstrings and inner thighs, too. The sumo squat can be performed with a barbell, with dumb-bells above your shoulders or hanging between your legs, or holding the barbell between your legs.

Good Morning Sumo Squat

This move combines the butt-building benefits of the sumo squat with the glute activation of the good morning. To perform, pick up a dumbbell and hold it close to your chest. Set your feet wider than shoulder-width apart in preparation for a sumo squat. As you lower down into your squat, lean forward into a good morning. You'll end up in a wide squat position, leaning slightly forward. Engage and lift from your glutes, squeezing as you rotate your torso backward and stand back up. This backward-leaning glute contraction really activates and builds your backside. Be careful to use good form with this exercise and protect your lower back by engaging your core and not overextending yourself.

Jump Squats

If you want to train like an NBA star or track athlete, you'll want to try this explosive move. The jump squat has many variations and options to keep it fresh and challenging. Jump squats can be as simple as squatting down and jumping up off the ground to as grueling as jumping through the squat while holding dumbbells, a barbell, a weighted ball, or wearing a weighted vest. Movement adjustments can also be used to change the emphasis and intensity. For example, partial squats can amp up the burn or be used in combination with full movements. The jump squat can be turned into a pencil squat by bringing your legs together as you jump upward and straightening your arms up in the air. Jump squats are a great exercise for increasing power.

Pencil Squat

If you're someone who gets confused about knowing what to do with your arms in a squat, this move is for you. The pencil squat is essentially a jump squat where you keep your arms overhead as you lower down and leap up. As you jump, to achieve the pencil line, bring both feet together and then spread them back out as you drop back down into the squat.

Triceps Extension Squat

The triceps extension squat is a compound movement well-suited for dumbbells or kettlebells. In addition to your booty, you'll give your triceps some TLC in this squat with arm extension. As you squat down, swing your arms slightly behind your hips, holding your weights in hand. As you stand up straight, extend your arms and swing the weights overhead. With your arms straight overhead, lower the weights down behind your head, keeping your upper arms straight as you perform a triceps extension.

Side-to-Side Squats

Side-to-side squats are a dynamic exercise where you leap or step back and forth laterally and then squat down after each sideways jump or step. To up the challenge, you can jump over an object and let your interior foot land or briefly touch its surface. With its bounce and give, a BOSU ball is a great tool to use with your side-to-side squats. Testing your agility and coordination, these side-to-side squats will force you to get lower and move more precisely as you tap each foot on the BOSU ball. This exercise is a different way to add in some core work, too. Throw on a weight vest or add some dumbbells to really burn your backside.

Deep Squat with Raised Heels

To perform the deep squat with raised heels, stand on your tiptoes and then lower into the squat position. Stay on your toes the whole time you exercise. This exercise will test your balance and coordination as much as your legs and glutes. The deep squat with heel raise is reminiscent of the chair pose in yoga. The heel raise will get your calves and quads burning, as well as your back and shoulders. If you want to make it more challenging, alternate heel raises or add weight. As a less balance-intensive alternative, you can also squat with raised heels with your heels elevated and supported on a small block, weight plate, or ledge.

. . .

Plie Squat with Toe Raise

The plie squat with toe lift is a variation on the goblin squat with a toe raise. To perform the plie squat with toe lift, stand with your legs slightly wider than shoulder-width apart and position your feet angled outward at about 45° while holding a weight in front of your chest with your elbows held close to your body. Drop down into a deep squat, keeping the weight in front of your chest and pointing your elbows to the insides of your knees. Stand up powerfully, lifting up onto your toes as you extend your legs while keeping your knees soft. Lower back down into the squat and repeat.

Pop Squat

The pop squat is an explosive, plyometric squat where you cross your legs as you jump into the air. To pop those squats, stand tall with your feet wider than shoulder-distance apart. Squat down, bending your knees 90° or more, and lower your hands toward the floor. The lower you go into your squat, the more of your hands will touch the ground. Pushing through your heels, explode off the floor. As you jump up into the air, cross your legs briefly. Uncross your legs before landing on soft knees. Return to the starting position and repeat, this time crossing the opposite leg in front. Increase the difficulty by adding weight like dumbbells or a weight vest, going deeper into the squat, or jumping higher.

Diagonal Squat Thrust

The diagonal squat thrust is a variation of the burpee where you jump your feet forward from a plank position and up into a squat with your hips squared to the front. You will then stand or jump up to a full upright position before lowering back down into a squat and hopping your legs back into the plank position. For more intensity, jump up into the air from the squat instead of jumping or stepping to a standing position. You can also use a weight vest or hold dumbbells in your hands as you jump to increase the difficulty.

. . .

Low Squat Walk / Monster Walk

Channel your inner prowling, stalking monster with low squat or monster walks. Low squat walks or monster walks are not to be confused with duck walks. The emphasis with squat walks is going down into a squat position and walking forward, backward, or to the side to light your glutes and quads on fire. Although monster walks are often demonstrated as primarily a lateral movement, the monsters prowling this book are not confined to side-to-side steps. To start your squat walks, stand with your feet hip-distance apart with your arms in front of your chest. Squat down, keeping your bodyweight over your heels. Step your left foot slightly out to the left, staying in a low squat. Bring your right foot up to meet your left. Step to the right side, bringing your left foot up to meet the right. Stay in the squat position while you work. Reverse the movements and repeat for your targeted steps, remaining in a low squat throughout the exercise. Step to the side and back to change the exercise emphasis, or freestyle and prowl in all directions—just don't scare the kids. Add difficulty by adding weight or bands, going lower, or staying down longer. Bands can also be looped around your thighs, by your knees, or at your ankles to alter the exercise angle, intensity, and emphasis.

Lateral Squat Walk / Side Lunge Walk

The side or lateral squat walk is the booty-building hybrid of a squat and lunge, or a sideways modified version of a monster walk. To perform, lower down into a squat or horse position and step out to the side. In this variation of the squat walk, your trailing leg will stay straight as you squat down and step out with your bent leading leg. Bring this trailing leg back up to return to the squatting position. Step to the side in one direction before going back to the other. For more glute activation, add bands around your thighs or hold something heavy in your arms, like dumbbells, kettlebells, a sandbag, or a nice, solid rock.

Cable Squat Walk-Outs

Throw in a cable machine with your low squat walks and you get the cable squat walk-out. Your backside won't know what hit it after this exercise. To start, attach either the rope handle or a straight bar handle at the lower end of the cable machine. The attachment does not need to be all the way at the bottom of the machine. Hold the cable attachment with extended arms and walk back a few steps away from the machine. Lower into a squat position and prepare for the fun to begin! While remaining in the squat, with a neutral spine and lifted chest, take six steps backwards followed by six steps forward. Keep the weight in your heels when you take each step to allow for maximum glute engagement, and make sure your knees don't collapse inwards. Each cycle back and forward together counts for one repetition. Add more weight or reps to boost the burn.

Wall Ball Shot

The wall ball shot is a CrossFit® staple. Basically, you take a heavy medicine ball, squat down, and propel the ball up into the air against the wall as you explode up into a standing position. You then catch the ball as you lower to repeat. To do your wall ball shots, find a good high solid wall. Start with your feet about shoulder-width apart. Hold the medicine ball at your chest. Brace your core. Lower your hips back and down. At the bottom, your hips should be lower than your knees. Maintain proper back alignment in your lumbar curve. Your knees should track above your toes throughout the movement. Your elbows should not touch your knees as you drop. Extend your hips and legs rapidly upward, throwing the ball at a target on the wall as you extend up and out. Keep your heels down on the floor until your hips and legs extend. Catch the ball and lower smoothly into the next rep.

Figure Four Squat

Part yoga, part squat, and all gains, the figure four squat is an excellent booty builder. Begin from a standing position with your feet roughly hip-distance apart. Balancing on your right leg, cross your left ankle up onto the lower part of your right thigh, just above the knee. Bend your right knee and squat as low as you can. If you can, target a 90° angle with your knee. Straighten your leg back up to a standing position. Repeat for your targeted reps, trying to stay balanced and controlled throughout. Switch sides and repeat with your other leg. Add weights, go lower, slow the movement down, or hold at the bottom of the squat to make the exercise harder.

The squat is one of the most effective whole-body exercises out there. Luckily for your glutes, the squat is great for them too. While this is a fairly comprehensive sample of squatting exercises, there's always room for more. Go activate those glutes, try out these exercises, and discover more!

LUNGING EXERCISES

Lunges combine strength, balance, and coordination in a dynamic addition to your lower-body workout. While squats have a broader base of support, the split stance in lunges forces you to constantly re-adjust your weight and muscle engagement. They can also challenge your mobility, balance, and stability, putting your hip, foot, and ankle stability to the test. From plyometrics to laterals to curtsies, lunge variations fire up your glutes, quads, thighs, and calves for superior leg strength. As an added benefit, lunges can be performed in any direction to hit your glutes from multiple angles. Lunges are also a great base or complement to other exercises to create compound, multijoint exercises to work the whole body.

Basic or Traditional Lunges

A lunge is performed by going up and down from a split-legged position with one foot forward and the other back. You can step into and out of lunges—forward or backward—or remain in the lunge position with one leg forward and the other back as you straighten your legs. As you lunge, you can keep your weight centered and balanced or shift it forward or backward as you exercise. You can keep your back leg straight or bent to adjust the points of exertion as you work. With lunges, you can adjust your leg positions, step and exertion angles, and rate of exertion. Lunges can be deep or shallow, performed from front to back or side to side or at a diagonal, with or without weights or other forms of resistance, and incorporate other movements. Because the lunge is a dynamic, flexible move performed over a wide range of motions, the variations are endless. Below are some examples of the many possible permutations on the basic lunge.

Sprinter Lunges

If you've ever watched sprinters or hurdlers on the track, you probably seen them performing sprinter lunges while warming up and training. The sprinter lunge improves power and pumps up your glute muscles as you work. The sprinter lunge is also perfect to practice working on your coordination as you drive your opposite arm to your opposite knee as you drive up. Try for height, not distance, with each step. To begin, stand tall with your feet shoulder-width apart. Step your left leg back into a reverse lunge, going as low as you can while keeping your back straight and making sure to maintain a bend in both legs. Hold at the bottom of this lunge position and then push through your right heel to explode up, driving the left knee forward and up. Try to get your working leg as high as possible before returning to the starting lunge position. Complete all reps with one leg, or change things up and alternate between legs in an exaggerated forward high-knee walk.

Plyometric Lunges

Plyometrics—explosive leaping or jump training—combined with lunges creates an exceptionally effective booty blaster and leg builder. Plyometric lunges can be as simple as jumping into the air and switching your feet forward and back when you're off the ground to as challenging as weighted jumps while doing HIIT training. Plyometric lunges can be performed with just about any lunge variation. Raising alternate arms as you jump turns the plyometric lunge into a split jack, a variation of the jumping jack.

• • •

Side Jump Lunge

The side jump lunge is a variation of the plyometric lunge where you skip or jump out to the side into a side lunge. Begin standing with your feet about hip-distance apart. Lunge to your right side, bending your right knee about 90° while keeping your left leg straight. Keeping your left knee aligned with your toes, push your glutes out behind you. Jump up, shifting your weight to the left. Land with your left knee bent and your right leg out to the side, bending your left knee about 90°. Repeat until your booty burns. Add weight, more reps, or bigger jumps to increase the difficulty.

Plyometric Lunges with Figure Eights

If you think plyo lunges are challenging, get ready to up the ante with plyometric lunges with figure eights. To perform these lunges, get a ball—a basketball, tennis ball, baseball, or football will do. While you jump into the air, loop the ball under and between your legs, switching the ball from one hand to the other. Jump again and switch the direction the ball moves between your legs and which leg is forward. These plyo lunges double-team coordination and endurance in one dynamic move.

Drummer Lunges with Battle Ropes

Drummer lunges with battle ropes are exactly what they sound like. Imagine you're drumming in the air, arms moving up and down except you're not drumming, you're moving heavy weighted battle ropes up and down. While your arms work the ropes, step backward into alternating reverse lunges. This move is great for taking out aggression and elevating your heart rate. Reverse lunges with battle ropes get your arms moving, increase your heart rate, and blast you with a full-body burn. They're pretty good for stress relief, too.

Parallette Lunges

Parallette lunges are performed by resting the top of one of your feet on or over low parallel bars. Parallette lunges are a bit like Bulgarian squats except your foot hinges on top of the bar and the lunge is typically broader with your feet wider apart than in Bulgarian squats. Like Bulgarian squats, using parallette bars gives your lunges some incline so you can improve the depth and intensity of the movement. You can also work with a pair of dumbbells or a set of bands to add some weight for an even better butt lift.

Lateral / Side Lunge to Clean

A lateral lunge is simply a lunge performed to the side. A clean is bringing a weight up to your chest—in this case a pair of kettlebells or dumbbells. Lateral lunges to clean are a great way to move and work in more than one plane of motion. This complex combination exercise will help you break outside the traditional exercise box and move dynamically. Be sure to recruit your glutes, hamstrings, and core—the less you use your arms, the more you'll work your glutes—to pop the pair of kettlebells up to chest height before dropping the weight back down between your legs as you lunge to the side.

Lunge to Plyo Hop

Relive your childhood joy of bouncing and flying through the air with this exciting lunge. Placing your front leg on a mini-trampoline and your back leg behind you, press down onto the trampoline with your front leg and bounce into the air. As you lift upward, raise your back leg off the ground to really crunch your glutes. The trampoline adds fun—and extra height—to basic plyo lunges. If you don't have a mini-tramp or other suitable launching pad, use a BOSU ball, step, low wall, or box.

Diagonal Lunge A-Step

Combining skipping over a box—or other suitable stable object—with a diagonal lateral lunge, the diagonal lunge A-step is a true physical challenge. To perform this compound exercise, hop up onto and over a low box. Your feet will touch the surface only briefly as you skip over the box. As both feet return to the ground, bring your inside leg back and across behind your body into a diagonal lunge. For stability, you can bring one hand down onto the box as you lunge back. Repeat on the other side to complete the exercise circuit, alternating back and forth on each side. Combining strength and speed, this box jump lunge will help improve your agility and endurance. A true calorie scorcher, the diagonal lunge A-step exercise will make you engage your abs and arms to help you jump onto the box as you start to lose steam. The bigger the movement, the better the burn—and potential results.

Overhead Lunges with Weights

If you want to work your shoulders, arms, and abs while building your backside, try overhead lunges with weights. Press a weight overhead—dumbbells, kettlebells, a slam ball, a laundry bag or basket, a sandbag, a sleeping cat, or whatever else works—while lunging. Hold the weights overhead while you lunge. To change the move up, you can press the weights up and down while you lunge to add intensity. Add plyometric lunges to increase the calorie burn as you press the weights overhead. These forward lunges will strengthen every facet of your booty. As an added bonus, holding resistance overhead also sculpts your abs and arms.

Step Ups

The step up is one of the best butt-building exercises you can do to focus on strength, power, and balance in a unilateral fashion, one side at a time. To perform a step up, stand with your right foot on a platform such as a bench or step, holding dumbbells by your sides with your arms straight—or start with your left foot if you're so inclined. Push upward through your right heel and step up onto the platform with both feet. Finally, step down to the floor with your right foot first, then left. Try to focus your efforts in your working leg to really isolate and build your glutes. For a bit of variation, push your non-lifting leg back to clench the other side of your buttocks as you push up off the ground. Step ups can be performed sequentially, stepping up with the same leg until your set is complete or alternating legs between steps.

Step Up and Lift

The step up and leg lift is an effective booty-building variation on the step up. To do the step up with leg lift, stand to one side of a flat bench, sturdy platform, or box. Place your right foot on the support in preparation to step up with your knee bent at 90 degrees while holding dumbbells or kettlebells at your sides. Step up onto the bench, pushing through your right leg until it is fully extended. Simultaneously, lean forward as you lower your weight to mid-shin while lifting your left leg to hip height behind you, parallel to the floor. Lower your left foot back to the floor while keeping your right foot on the bench. Throw on a weight vest, hold dumbbells, or add ankle weights or bands to add more booty-building challenge.

Step Rainbow or Half-Moon
The step rainbow or half-moon involves shifting the angles of your step backs after stepping up onto a platform to work your glutes from multiple angles. To perform the step rainbow or step half-moon, stand toward the back of a bench, box, or other stable platform. Bending your left knee, step off the platform to the right side, tapping your right toes on the ground and keeping your weight mostly over your left leg. Stand up on the platform, then step your right leg behind the bench to the left side, touching down with your toes. Straighten your left leg and return to the starting position. Continue for your desired repetitions before switching sides. To make the step more challenging, hold dumbbells, slow down, or move to a higher step or bench.

Step Hop with Reverse Lunge
The step hop combines a dynamic plyo step with a deep lunge to strengthen your legs and backside. Start standing behind a bench, low box, or other sturdy platform. Place your left foot flat on the elevated surface. Step or pop up onto the bench, bringing your right knee to about hip height like you're doing an elevated, extended sprint. Step back to the starting position, then bring your left foot behind you into a reverse lunge, bending both knees 90°. Step back to the starting position and repeat. To add difficulty, pop up onto the bench, use weights, or bands.

. . .

Cable Alternating Step Ups

The cable step up is a variation of the basic step up using a cable machine instead of weights. To start, place a box or bench in front of a cable machine. Ideally, you want the platform to be at a height where your thigh is parallel to the ground when you set your foot on the elevated surface. Attach a single handle to each side of the cable machine on the bottom setting and hold one in each hand. With your arms extended while holding the cables, step up onto the bench starting with the foot of your weaker leg. Keep your spine neutral and your chest up as you work. Push up through the middle of your foot until you are standing on top of the bench. Finish with both feet on the bench. Step back down with the same foot you stepped up with first. Begin your next repetition with the opposite foot. As an alternative, do this exercise leading with one leg at a time before switching to the other leg and doing all your reps with that leg. More weight, a higher step, and slower, controlled movements will add more difficulty.

Stairs, Hills, or Stair Machine

Walking and running can be thought of as modified moving lunges. Walking or running up hills or stairs or on a stair machine are phenomenal ways to engage your glutes and work on your cardio. As you walk or run, be sure to engage your glutes and contract those muscles. As much as possible, try to drive from your glutes to get the maximum effort from your muscles as you walk or run. Finding a nice stairwell at work can be a perfect place to take a break and build your backside while incorporating exercise into your day-to-day routine.

Split Jacks

Split jacks are a variation of the jumping jack where you jump with your feet forward and backward instead of side-to-side as you would in a normal jumping jack. As you leap, raise one arm into the air, alternating arms as you jump. In a split jack, you will use your arms differently than in plyometric lunges, tending to bounce more than leap, and you won't spread your feet quite as far apart as in the plyo lunge to help with your jumps. But both motions are very similar and can be argued to be variations on a single movement.

Predator Split Jacks

Predator split jacks are a variation of the split jack where you bring both arms straight out to the side and then behind you as you jump back with one leg. Jumping back to the center with both feet beneath you, bring your arms together straight out in front of you. This move turns up the cardio while building strength in your lower body. This split jack variation uses your arms, shoulders, and back to help you create maximum force and build your booty.

Pendulum Lunge

The pendulum lunge is a bit like the plyometric lunge with figure eight except without the ball and the jumping is optional. In a controlled manner, as you step into a forward lunge, lean forward when your front foot plants on the ground. When your torso touches your thigh, bring both hands together to clap between your legs. The pendulum lunge lets you slow things down to tone things up. The pendulum lunge takes balance to a new level as your gluteus maximus works overtime to help stabilize your stance while you change positions and alter your center of gravity.

Curtsy Lunge

To do a curtsy lunge, grab a small towel, rolled shirt, or band in your hands and hold it taut out in front of you. While holding the towel or band straight, step backward and across your body into a deep curtsy. This is a curtsy lunge. The towel is optional, but the burn is not. Curtsy lunges may look like a basic dance move, but these butt burners also sculpt your inner thighs and quads as well. Holding the towel tightly also strengthens your core and arms. Substitute a dumbbell for the towel for an added challenge. As a more difficult, butt-building variation, try not to let your back leg touch the ground, let your foot glide on the floor, or only let the top of your foot touch the ground as it angles out behind you in the lunge.

Lateral Lunge with Burpee Walkout

Burpees are a complex, compound movement to start. The lateral lunge with burpee walkout brings this complexity and butt burn to a new level. Start by performing a lateral lunge to one side. When you bring your foot back beneath your shoulders after the lateral lunge, go into a deep squat, lowering your bottom and hands toward the ground. As your hands touch the floor, walk your feet out from the squat into a plank. Bring your feet back up into a low squat, stand, and begin the motion on the other side with a lateral lunge on your other leg. Amp up the intensity by jumping or hopping from move to move or adding a weight vest. This exercise is a great way to improve functional movements and add them into your training.

Cable Reverse Lunges

Reverse lunges are a great glute developer. Reverse lunges with a cable machine add an exciting twist on this booty classic. Begin by attaching a rope handle to the bottom of the cable machine. Stand with your back towards the cable machine. Duck under the cable so that the rope handle is behind your head and your hands are just above each of your shoulders. Walk the cable out away from the machine to give yourself enough space to drop into a reverse lunge. Stand with your feet shoulder-width apart to begin the movement. Take a long step backward into a reverse lunge, bending both knees and lowering yourself towards the ground. Keep your chest up and your weight in the heel of your front foot during the lunge. Step forward, back into the starting position. Repeat on the same leg for the desired number of repetitions.

The lunge is, at its core, a simple exaggerated step. But, step by exaggerated step, lunges will help you develop the glutes of your dreams. Don't neglect lunges on your path to glute mastery!

DEADLIFTS AND RELATED HINGING EXERCISES

Deadlifts are an ideal hinging movement to really work those buttocks as you clench and flex your glutes while you lift up and then slowly lower weights down to the floor, really engaging your muscles. As an added bonus, deadlifts work your hamstrings and lower back to strengthen your entire posterior chain. In addition to boosting your backside aesthetics, deadlifts develop your glute and hamstring strength and power. Together, these muscles contribute to nearly every athletic movement, including sprinting and jumping, but, beyond athletics, having strong glutes, hamstrings, and lower back will help you navigate life with strength and stability—a goal we should all aspire to achieve.

Form is critical with deadlifts and should always be monitored since poor form will put undue pressure on your back, especially with heavy weights. Also, keep your back straight—no rounding—and hinge at the hips. Exercising barefoot or in socks can help with stability and weight engagement as you connect with the floor. If you're lifting heavy, straps to assist your grip will help you focus on working the primary muscles you're engaging —your glutes—before other muscles you're not working on fail or limit your efforts (e.g., your grip).

. . .

Traditional Deadlift

The deadlift or traditional deadlift is a simple exercise that can be very challenging to execute properly, especially as weight—and ego—increase. When picking up your weight—dumbbells, kettlebells, bands, or barbells —from the floor, assume a squat-like position with a straight back. Drive up through your legs and glutes; do not pull up with your back. Contract through your hamstrings and glutes as you lift and straighten into a standing position. Clench your buttocks to help finish the move and accentuate the glutes at the top. From the standing position, hinge forward at the waist, keeping your back straight. As you lower, extend your buttocks outward behind you to counterbalance the weight held in your hands and reduce pressure on your back. Try to keep the focus of your exertion in your glutes as you descend.

If you've never deadlifted before, perform a few practice lifts without weights to get a feel for the exercise and find the proper form. You'll know you're close when you feel the exertion in your hamstrings along the backs of your legs and up into your glutes but not in your lower back. For those who are less flexible, you may not be able to lower your dumbbells or barbell all the way to the floor. As your strength and flexibility increase, you can increase the range of your movement. But, again, always avoid putting the focus of the work in your back. To target the glutes further, you can restrict the deadlift movement so that you are working only in the top of the range of motion. For those with back issues, this limited range also helps protect the lower back.

Stiff Leg Deadlift

The stiff leg deadlift is performed like a conventional deadlift except you keep your legs straightened throughout the movement, avoiding knee bend. To do a stiff leg deadlift, stand with your feet shoulder-width apart, holding a barbell or dumbbell in an overhand grip (i.e., with your palms facing you). Your knees should be no more than slightly bent—the aim is to maintain this slight degree of flex throughout the movement. Bend at your hips and lower the barbell, keeping your back straight. Lower until you feel the stretch in your hamstrings and glutes, and then slowly straighten back up. Maintain the bar or weights close to your body throughout and avoid jerky movements—keep the exercise slow and controlled.

Sumo Deadlift

The sumo deadlift is performed using an extra-wide stance that changes the lifting orientation and the primary muscles used in the dead-lift. Because your legs are wide—wider than shoulder-width—you will not lean forward as much as in a traditional deadlift as you lift the weight up. This change in orientation means the lower back doesn't work as hard while the hips, hamstrings, and quads pick up the slack. The sumo deadlift is a great way to improve mobility—a benefit not often associated with heavy lifts. To establish your base, angle your feet outward slightly between roughly sixty and forty-five degrees. This will force you to keep your knees out as you drive the weight up. To really get your glutes firing while doing your sumo deadlifts, try bending your knees slightly and holding them in this bent position to avoid lateral shifting as you lift. This will take your quads out of the exercise and really get your glutes squeezing to lift the weight. In this case, you'll rotate up, over, and around your hips as you lean back, lock in those glutes, and lift around your locked knees. Make sure your back is secure, stable, and safe as you lift. Consider resetting after each rep to make sure your form is good. Sumo deadlifts are great with both heavy and low weights as well as high reps and light weights. Both can be fantastic for your butt.

Deficit Deadlift

Deficit deadlifts involve standing on a small box, board, or plate to increase the distance the bar travels as you lower it down to the ground, allowing a greater range of motion in the lift. Picking up the bar from this position is more challenging—remember your back, so you won't be able to lift as much weight as in a traditional deadlift. However, this greater range of motion is a fantastic way to increase strength and even improve your conventional deadlifts.

Block Deadlift

Block deadlifts employ the opposite strategy from the deficit deadlift. With block deadlifts, you elevate the bar or weight on blocks, plates, or rack pins to reduce the range of the exercise motion. This limited range of motion allows you to lift more weight, challenges your nervous system, protects your back, and develops the top portion of your deadlift, the part that really hits your backside.

Dumbbell Deadlift

Dumbbell deadlifts are simply deadlifts performed with dumbbells. Since you probably won't be lifting as much weight as you would in a traditional deadlift with a bar—dumbbells generally aren't that heavy—you won't build maximum strength or gain as much mass. The dumbbell deadlift is, however, a great variation for learning the exercise, is easily accomplished at home, and will still allow you to grow and develop. You can also perform dumbbell deadlifts for high reps during conditioning circuits or as finishing exercises to build endurance in the muscles of your posterior chain—that's everything on the back side of your body.

Kettlebell Sumo Deadlift

Kettlebell sumo deadlifts are a great deadlift option, especially for those who want to build their backside from the comforts of home. While the kettlebell sumo deadlift's name implies similarities to a sumo deadlift, the movement is actually closer to a trap bar deadlift motion. Kettlebell sumo deadlifts are performed almost like a squat, with the weight in your hands. Because the weight is lighter and the movement allows you to maintain more of an upright torso than some other deadlifts, kettlebell sumo deadlifts are great for people with lower back issues who have problems with some other deadlift variations like barbell deadlifts. Kettlebell sumo deadlifts are an excellent exercise to start with before progressing to heavier barbell deadlift variations. They are also a nice exercise for more advanced lifters looking to do some higher rep work near the end of a workout.

Romanian Deadlift

The Romanian deadlift (RDL) is a variation of the conventional deadlift in which you start from a standing position—conventional deadlifts start from the floor—and sit your hips back and then lower the bar down your shins. As you start, you might not be able to touch the bar to the ground because of limited hamstring flexibility. If you want to target your glutes, you may not want the weights to touch the ground whether you're flexible enough for them to reach the floor or not. The Romanian deadlift shifts the focus of your lift from your lower back to your hamstrings and glutes. Given this glute and hamstring focus, Romanian deadlifts are a wonderful exercise for your booty.

Single-Leg Romanian Deadlift and Walking Single-Leg Romanian Deadlift

The single-leg Romanian deadlift is a fantastic, targeted booty-builder. You can use just about any weight with this exercise, from a mini barbell or dumbbell to a kettlebell or band. To start, stand with your feet hip-width apart, holding a kettlebell with one hand or a pair of dumbbells in both hands with your palms facing your thighs. Keeping your spine neutral and your feet and legs stable, hinge at the hips—bend at the waist while pushing your hips toward the wall behind you and allow the weight to lower toward your shins. As you lower the weight, bend your right knee slightly and lift your left leg out behind you to provide a counterbalance. Keep the weight in front of your forward, bending leg. Squeeze your glutes and press through your right heel to return to the standing position. Repeat on the same side to burn out those muscles before switching.

The single-leg Romanian deadlift is one of the best ways to eliminate muscle imbalances in your glutes and hamstrings on the left and right sides of your body. It also improves balance, stability, and core control. The single-leg Romanian deadlift can be turned into a walking single-leg Romanian deadlift by alternating working legs and stepping forward after each rep.

Landmine Romanian Deadlift

The landmine Romanian deadlift is an unheralded glute grower. This move hits both the working leg and the stabilizing one. To perform, use a landmine or a barbell braced against something stable. Hold the nonstationary end of the barbell in one hand. Lift one leg and lean forward, focusing on squeezing the glute to control the movement down and back up. The end of the barbell will drop as you hinge forward, and your glutes will begin to burn. Engage your glutes to lift back up to the starting position. Try not to tap your non-working leg to keep those stabilizing muscles firing. Add more weight for more challenge and gains.

Cable Romanian Deadlifts

The cable machine Romanian deadlift is a very effective non-traditional glute burner. Attach a straight bar handle to the cable machine on the bottom setting to start. Hold the bar with an overhand grip with your hands about shoulder-width apart. Walk the cable out and stand with your feet no wider than hip-width apart. The exercise begins from the standing position, holding the bar with extended arms and your weight resting in your heels. With a slight bend in your knees and a neutral spine, push your hips backwards while lowering your chest towards the floor. As you lower, extend the bar towards the cable machine to create a stretch through your hamstrings. Pull back up to the starting position using your hamstrings and glutes. Squeeze your glutes at the top before going down into the next repetition. For more muscle engagement, try single-leg cable Romanian deadlifts.

B-Stance Romanian Deadlift

The B-stance Romanian deadlift is a nice exercise that can be performed almost anywhere using your bodyweight on up. To start, stand with your feet hip-width apart, holding dumbbells at your sides with your palms facing inward. Line the front of your right foot up with the back of your left foot and lift your right heel off the floor. Keep the majority of the weight and exertion in the planted foot. Hinge forward from your hips, bringing your weights down toward the floor as you push your glutes behind you, feeling a stretch along your hamstrings. Keep your abs engaged and your back flat, forming a straight line from your head to your glutes. Straighten back up to the standing position, keeping your heel raised. Repeat for all your reps, and then switch legs and repeat.

Single-Leg Cable Deadlift

Combining the constant tension of the cable machine with the backside building of the deadlift, the single-leg cable deadlift is a functional exercise in any booty-building program. To perform your single-leg cable deadlift, attach a single handle to the bottom of the cable machine. Hold the cable with an extended arm in the hand that is opposite to the leg you're working. From a standing position with your feet close together, hinge forward at the hips. As you lean forward, keep one leg grounded while lifting the other out behind you and maintaining a neutral spine. Keep your core engaged and your feet firm to assist with balance. Let your hips act like a pivot—your chest only goes down as far as your back leg comes up. Try to get your back and floating leg parallel to the ground before engaging through the glute of your working leg and pulling back up to the starting position. Keep your repetitions slow and controlled. Do all your reps on one leg before changing sides.

Snatch-Grip Deadlift

The snatch-grip deadlift is a deadlift variation performed with any other deadlift by changing your grip from a narrow to wide position—the same broad grip employed in snatches. When you use an extra-wide grip, one wider than your shoulders, your back and traps work harder to hold the weight. With the wider grip, your reach is effectively shorter, so you also increase the range of motion of the exercise. In this way, the snatch-grip deadlift functions similarly to deficit deadlifts and can really target those glutes.

Trap Bar Deadlift

The trap bar—or hex bar—is an open bar that is curved around your body so that you lift from the center of mass as opposed to leaning forward over a conventional straight barbell. The trap bar deadlift is easier to perform than standard deadlifts because you stand in the middle of the weight instead of holding it in front of your body. This change in lifting orientation allows you to lift more, helps protect your back, and lets you focus your efforts on building your muscles, especially your glutes. Given the trap bar's versatility, you can perform almost all the deadlift variations with a trap bar, except those that require other equipment, like dumbbell deadlifts.

Cable Pull Throughs

Although not a traditional deadlift, cable pull throughs incorporate a similar, glute-focused movement with a cable machine. To start, attach a rope handle to the bottom of the cable machine. Hold one side of the rope handle in each hand and step over the cable so the cable is in between your legs. You should be facing away from the cable machine (i.e., your back will be toward the machine). Walk a few steps away from the cable machine to give yourself adequate space to work. Begin by standing straight up with the rope handle gripped with your arms extended down between your thighs. With a slight bend in your knees and a neutral spine, hinge at your hips, driving your glutes back and allowing your hands and the cable to go through your legs and out behind you. You should feel a stretch through your hamstrings. From this extended position, engage your glutes and pull back up to a standing position, giving your buttocks a solid squeeze at the top of the movement. To avoid giving yourself too much time to rest and recover, don't pause too long at the top before beginning your next repetition.

· · ·

Kettlebell Swings

Kettlebell swings are not a traditional deadlift exercise, but they take the driving and hinging motions of a deadlift and combine them with the explosive movements of a plyometric jump while engaging your core and shoulders in a whole-body glute builder. To perform kettlebell swings, stand tall, gripping the kettlebell with two hands, letting the weight rest centered in front of your hips and legs. Keep your arms long and loose while squeezing your shoulder blades together and engaging your core. Soften your knees, shift your bodyweight into your heels, and lower your buttocks back and down behind you. Driving through your heels and glutes, explode forward and up through your hips to send the weight swinging upward from your quads. Aim for the kettlebell to reach roughly chest height with your arms extended. Achieving this finishing position requires you to snap your hips forward and through, contracting your core while squeezing your glutes. While the kettlebell begins to descend, let the weight do the work as you ready your body for the next rep. As the kettlebell drops, shift your weight back into your heels while hinging at your hips and loading both your hamstrings and glutes. Receive the weight of the kettlebell through your legs and glutes, allowing the weight to swing back between your legs. As the kettlebell makes the transition from backward to forward, drive up and through your heels, glutes, and hips to repeat.

Good Mornings

Good mornings are an excellent glute and hamstring exercise performed simply by bending forward at the waist with weight, for example holding a barbell at your shoulders or against your chest. Good mornings can be thought of as the top portion of a deadlift. To perform, lean forward, keeping your chest up, and shift your hips and glutes back. Bend until your torso is parallel to the floor but no farther. Clench your buttocks and hamstrings to lift yourself back up to the starting position. More weight equals more gains. Perform your good mornings from a standing or seated position.

. . .

Banded Good Mornings

Like weighted good mornings, banded good mornings are great buttocks developers. Start from a standing position on the exercise band and loop the other end over the back of your shoulders and stand tall. Keeping your lower back in its natural arch, bend your hips back and lower your torso until it's nearly parallel to the floor. Keep your chest up and pointing forward as you work. Explosively extend your hips and drive through your glutes to come back up. Banded good mornings are a nice deadlift variation that can be easily performed at home.

Jefferson Deadlift / Jefferson Squat

The Jefferson deadlift—sometimes called the Jefferson squat—is a modified deadlift performed while straddling a barbell with the bar running between your legs. To do a Jefferson deadlift, straddle the barbell with your feet shoulder-width or slightly wider apart, grab the bar directly beneath your shoulders, and stand up. Make sure the weight is centered between both feet, and don't let your knees turn inward when you start pulling. Lower the weight straight back down without leaning forward as much as possible. While you can use different grips as you lift, stay relatively balanced by alternating your front and back foot for equal amounts of reps. One way to do this is to alternate which leg is forward during each set. As is the case with the trap bar deadlift, the Jefferson deadlift should be closer to a squat than a hinge. If you're leaning forward in a hinging motion, this can reduce your leverage.

Bending over and picking things up may be a chore at home, but in the gym or when done properly at home, these deadlifts will help you build the buttocks of your dreams.

GLUTE BRIDGES, HIP THRUSTS, LEG CURLS, AND LEG LIFTS

Not a fan of squats, deadlifts, and lunges? Glute bridges—raising your hips off the floor while your shoulders stay grounded or supported on an object—and their variations like hip thrusts are among the best booty sculptors around. By squeezing your glutes at full hip extension—when your body forms a diagonal line from your shoulders to your knees or a straight line when you lift your hips up off the ground while your shoulders are supported—you engage all three major muscles that make up your backside. Leg lifts work similar magic, but with balance thrown in. Because form is so crucial to getting the most out of each bridge and lift, it's best to nail down proper form before you get creative with your workouts. Glute bridges, hip thrusts, and leg lifts have the added benefit of working your posterior chain, so you work your backside while working your back.

Double-Leg Glute Bridge

Double-leg glute bridge are a booty-building staple. With both feet and your back resting on the floor, lift your hips up into the air as high as you can. Your body will form a triangle as your starting position. This exercise is great for building both your glutes and lower back. Double-leg glute bridges are so good that they're not only a booty-building fundamental, but a physical therapy staple for lower back strengthening and recovery. To add additional intensity, rest weights like dumbbells or a barbell on your hips as you exercise. As the weights get heavier, you may want to add a cushion or towel to protect your hips and stomach. Whatever you do, glute bridges will sculpt your backside!

Hip Thrusts

Hip thrusts—sometimes called hip thrusters—are similar to double-leg glute bridges except your shoulders are up off the ground on a support with hip thrusters instead of on the ground as they are with glute bridges. With both feet and your back resting on a box, platform, bench, or other suitable support, drive through your feet as you lift your hips up into the air as high as you can. Like glute bridges, thrusts are amazing for building both your glutes and your lower back. Because your shoulders are elevated with your body forming an L-shape, you will have greater range of motion in the hip thruster relative to the glute bridge. For more difficulty and booty gains, rest a barbell or dumbbells on your hips. As the weights get heavier, you may want to add cushions or towels to protect your hips, stomach, and shoulders. Adjusting the direction of your feet (e.g., pointing your toes slightly outward) will also help you keep the focus of the exercise in your glutes instead of your hamstrings. Be sure to keep your back straight to reduce injury risks. For an even greater challenge, add glute bands—booty bands or basic bands—around your thighs that force your knees inward to your barbell hip thrusts. Resisting the inward pull of the bands while you thrust upward with the weight of the barbell will add glute gains from all angles, especially if you drive your knees outward against the band. Whatever you do, hip thrusts will help your glutes grow and improve your explosive, athletic potential!

Single-Leg Glute Bridge and Single-Leg Hip Thrusters

Single-leg glute bridges and hip thrusters are performed just like double-leg glute bridges and hip thrusters except you lift one leg up in the air as you work. Single-leg hip thrusters and glute bridges add an extra challenge to the exercise by not only making your work harder but by recruiting additional stability muscles to maintain good form. Small pulses in the elevated bridged position mean big gains for your booty. Your glutes will work extra hard to maintain balance while you fully extend your hips and leg. Be sure to keep your shoulders connected to the ground or your support to help stabilize your body. Weights like a dumbbell, barbell, or kettlebell will really add to the gains!

Suspension Trainer Single-Leg Glute Bridge

Suspension trainer single-leg glute bridges are a great way to work the whole range of gluteus muscles, given the instability incorporated into the movement. To perform, attach the suspension trainer to a sturdy overhead object and lengthen one handle to about knee height. Lie on your back on the floor and place the heel of your left foot in the foot cradle of the trainer. Bend your left knee about 90 degrees and extend your right leg straight out on the floor. Brace your abs and contract your glutes to bridge your hips off the floor while simultaneously lifting your right leg into the air until your right leg is in line with your left thigh. As you struggle to lift and remain stable, remember that all the hard work is for a better booty!

Suspension Trainer Glute Bridge

The suspension trainer glute bridge takes both of your feet off the ground, so you'll feel like you're flying as you work your glutes. To perform the suspension trainer glute bridge, set up as you would for the single-leg glute bridge, but rest both feet in the suspended foot cradles. Drive up through your heels to raise your hips off the floor to blast your booty. Try to keep your body stable to engage all your gluteus muscles as you lift and fly to those glute gains!

Cook Hip Lift

Performed like a single-leg glute bridge except you pull your non-working leg toward your chest instead of holding it out or pushing it up, the Cook hip lift—named after its creator, physical therapist Gray Cook—is another great butt lifter. To begin, lie face up on the floor and pull your left knee up to your chest. Hug your thigh tightly to your chest. Bend the right leg and plant your foot on the floor close to your buttocks. Drive through the middle of your foot and squeeze your glutes as you bridge your hips up—as with other bridges, they won't go high—until your hamstrings start to tense. Work to shift the tension into your glutes as you work. Repeat on both sides.

Bridge Abduction

The bridge abduction is a variation of the glute bridge that combines a bridge (lifting your hips up) and abduction (moving your legs away from the center of your body). Bridge abductions can be performed with double legs as you push your knees outward while your hips are elevated, or with a single leg as you lift one leg away from your body while your hips are up. This hip abduction is all about small, controlled movements. Pressing your shoulder blades and your standing foot into the floor creates a strong base. Adding bands looped around your knees or thighs will increase the difficulty, as will extending the time you hold your hips up off the ground.

Leaning Hip Abduction

The leaning hip abduction is another abduction variation to work the outsides of your glutes. To begin, kneel on the floor a few inches to the left of a stability ball, chair, bench, or other suitable support. Place your right elbow and forearm on the center of the support and your left hand on your hip. Extend your left leg diagonally to the side, forming a straight line from your shoulder to heel. Keeping your upper body still, lift your leg to hip height. Hold for one count, then lower your leg without touching the floor. Repeat for all your reps and then switch sides. To add more difficulty, add ankle weights or bands, increase your hold time, or raise your leg higher.

Squatting Abduction

This glute burner can be performed anywhere. To perform squatting abductions, lower into a squatting position with your feet slightly wider than shoulder-width apart—think of a sumo squat or horse stance. From this squatting position, push your knees outward and then bring them back in. For more of a challenge, add bands around your thighs, but you probably won't need them. Try to concentrate the work in your glutes as much as possible.

Hip Raises with Foam Roller

Hip raises with a foam roller are performed by resting your feet or one foot on a foam roller while you lift your hips. Try not to let the foam roller move while you lift your hips from the floor. In this exercise, the unstable tube underfoot forces you to squeeze and activate your glutes and your abs to reach full extension and maintain balance. With consistent exercise and a stronger lower back, you may not need the roller to help relax your back!

Reverse Table-Up

Tables might not have great glutes, but you can if you do reverse table-ups and its variations (e.g., single-legged table-ups, elevated table-ups, and weighted table-ups). To do reverse table-ups, sit on the floor and place your hands on the floor under your shoulders with your fingers pointing in front of you. Place your feet shoulder-width apart so that your legs will go up perpendicular to the floor. Squeeze your glutes to lift up off the floor. Push through your heels as you bridge your hips up. Your body should form a table with your torso and hips parallel to the floor. Hold for two seconds before lowering. Repeat for your desired number of reps. Add extra time or a weight vest for more of a challenge.

Bridge Tap Hollow Hold

The bridge tap hollow hold combines a Pilates stomach burner with a booty-lifting bridge. Simply perform a double or single-leg bridge. When your back returns to the ground, lift both feet off the floor. Simultaneously, hollow and round your chest as you lift your arms and shoulders from the floor. Extend your arms up and out behind you, and do the same with your feet and legs in front of you. This move lets your abs join in the body-building fun.

Chair Crunch and Butt Lift

The chair crunch and butt lift is another exercise that combines booty and belly benefits. While lying on your back on the floor with your feet resting up on a box, chair, or bench, lift upward with one or both legs, raising your hips off the ground. As you lift, you can tilt your foot up so that only your heel remains on the support or keep the whole bottom of your foot supported. After you lower yourself down and your back rests on the floor, perform a crunch. Repeat. This compound exercise strengthens your pelvic floor and core in addition to your glutes. Add a weighted vest or increase the height of your foot for more difficulty.

Prone Leg Lift / Hands and Knees Leg Lift

Lying on the floor on your stomach, lift one or both of your legs up into the air behind you. Be sure to contract your glutes as much as possible as you lift. Bands or ankle weights will add additional intensity, as will pulses at full extension and height. For more range of motion and booty-building potential, perform your leg lifts from your hands and knees—see quadruped hip extensions below for another variation.

Reverse Back Extension

Take your booty-building to another level with stability ball assisted back extensions. To perform, lie face-down on an exercise ball and walk your body forward until the ball supports your hips only, while resting your hands on the floor. Squeeze your glutes and raise your legs up behind you until they're level with your torso. Add ankle weights, pulses, bands, or more height to increase the difficulty.

Fire Hydrant / Side Leg Lift

The fire hydrant is a simple but effective booty builder. To perform, start in a quadruped position—on your hands and knees—with your wrists stacked directly under your shoulders and your hips over your knees. Keep your belly button drawn in toward your spine, your back flat, and your legs bent at 90 degrees. Lift one of your legs out to your side, stopping at hip height. Return to the starting position. That's one rep. If you've ever seen a pup visiting a fire hydrant, you'll have a pretty good idea how to perform this glute-building exercise. Change the angle of your leg lift or add weights or bands for more booty-building intensity.

Plank Leg Lift

To perform a plank leg lift, get in a stable plank position with your arms straight and your palms on the ground. Alternatively, bend your arms and let your forearms rest on the ground in a sphinx position. Keeping one leg straight with the ball of your foot resting on the ground, lift your leg up and out away from your body. In this three-legged plank, be sure to squeeze your glutes as you lift one leg off the ground, lift it up behind you, and/or tap it out to the side. Ankle weights or bands can add additional butt-building intensity.

Long Leg Marches

Imagine you're lying on your back on the floor, marching in place with your hips elevated off the ground. This is the buttocks and hamstring-building long leg march. To perform, lie down on the ground on your back. Bend your knees slightly. Rest both arms on the floor alongside your body for support. With your knees slightly bent, lift your legs and hips up off the ground. Your weight should be supported by your heels and your shoulders/upper torso. Now, slowly lift one leg up into the air and lower it back to the ground like you're marching in place. Alternate legs as you march in place on the floor while building your butt with every step.

Bird Dog Leg Lift / Super Dog Leg Lift

The bird dog leg lift is a dynamic variation of the hands and knees leg lift. However, instead of just lifting one leg, you lift an arm as well. To perform the bird dog leg lift, raise one leg up while resting on your hands and knees. Simultaneously, lift the arm diagonal to the elevated leg off the floor. This will leave you balancing on one leg and one arm as you extend your other arm forward and upward while lifting your other leg backward and upward.

Turn the bird dog into a super dog by sitting back and down onto the foot of your bent supporting leg. This will bring your torso much closer to the ground as you fold over. Hold your non-working arm bent down beside your chest for support. Keep your working leg and arm extended out in front and behind you while resting on the floor. Lift the extended leg and arm up off the ground to engage your glutes and shoulder. Your torso will remain resting on your bent leg while your glutes and shoulder work. The more you lift, the harder you work.

Half-Moon or Rainbow Leg Lifts

To perform half-moon or rainbow leg lifts, get on your hands and knees on the floor. Extend one leg straight behind you with a flexed foot. Describe an arch with your straightened leg, going from straight behind you and then up into the air and out to the side. Your leg will outline a semicircle like a half-moon or rainbow. Keeping your foot flexed when tapping the floor will help you engage your butt muscles more. Just a few reps are all you need to feel the burn for this floor exercise. To make the exercise more difficult, begin on a weight bench or other elevated surface for a greater range of motion, add ankle weights or bands, slow the motion down, and / or increase your rep range.

Glute Bridge with Foot Tap or Leg Lift

A glute bridge with foot tap or leg lift starts with both feet on the ground while you lie on the ground on your back. Then, lift your pelvis up in the air. As your hips reach the top of the movement, bring one leg up off the ground. Let your foot briefly tap the ground before repeating the motion. Perfect for beginners, this glute bridge helps you get used to balancing weight on one leg for a moment before bringing your foot back down. Remember to keep your butt lifted as you alternate sides.

Glute Bridge with Chest Press

The glute bridge with chest press is a compound exercise that combines both a glute bridge and a chest press. Lying on your back with your feet on the ground, lift your bottom up into the air to perform a bridge. As you raise your pelvis, simultaneously press the weights up off the ground and straighten your arms. This exercise is a great way to work on your total-body strength with low impact and build your backside.

Frog Pump / Frog Bridge

The frog pump is a variation of the double-leg glute bridge, except you keep your feet pressed together instead of directly below your knees as you work. With both feet and your back resting on the floor, bring the sides —or soles—of your feet together and lift your hips up into the air as high as you can. Your body will form a triangle above the ground and your legs will form a diamond as your feet stay pressed together. Like other bridges, this exercise is great for building both your glutes and your lower back. To add additional intensity, rest weights like dumbbells or a barbell on your hips as you exercise, go for more height, or hold the lift longer. To increase abductor activation, add bands around your thighs to make pressing your legs apart more difficult.

Hamstring Curl / Floor Sliders / Gliders

Your biceps aren't the only body part that benefits from curls! Your hamstrings and glutes do as well. Hamstring curls will literally lift your buns—and your buns will literally lift if you keep working—with this intense exercise. Hamstring curls use a stability ball, gliders, a folded towel, or even socks on a smooth surface to work your glutes, hamstrings, and core. Sliding hamstring curls are sometimes called slick floor curls or slick bridge curls and are not just for fun and enjoyment. Begin by lying face-up with your legs straight and your heels pressed into the top of the stability ball, gliders, or towel with your arms extended by your sides. Pressing through your glutes, lift your lower back a few inches off the floor. Pull your heels toward your glutes, lifting your hips a few inches higher as you pull. Roll or slide back to extend your legs to return to the starting position.

Stability Ball /Suspension Hamstring Curl / Hamstring Frog Curls

With one foot or both feet resting on an exercise ball, press up into a bridge, contracting your glutes and pulling with your hamstrings as you press up and pull the ball toward you. Play with which muscles are taking the brunt of the exercise to challenge yourself and hit where you want. As you lower, extend your feet back out to relax the curl. For even more of a challenge, try to do these hamstring curls with a suspension trainer. These hamstring curls take glute bridges and basic hamstring curls to the next level while strengthening your hamstrings as you fight for stability. The instability of the exercise ball challenges you to move in slow, controlled movements. If you perform this exercise with your knees out instead of straight up while curling, you're doing a hamstring frog curl.

Figurehead

If you want to strike a pose while building your glutes, the figurehead is perfect for you! To perform the figurehead, lie on the floor face down with your arms at your sides. Squeeze your glutes and raise your torso, arms, and legs simultaneously so that only your hips are touching the floor. Imagine reaching back and trying to touch your feet with your hands. Hold for a second at the top, then return to the starting position so your shoulders touch the floor.

Superman / Superwoman

If striking a pose isn't enough and you want to turn into a glute-building superhero, the superman / superwoman is your go-to exercise! To perform the superman, lie on the floor face down with your arms out in front of you. Squeeze your glutes and raise your torso, arms, and legs simultaneously so that only your hips are touching the floor. Imagine reaching out and flying through the air like Superman or Superwoman as you clench your glutes and tighten your lower back. Hold for a second at the top, then return to the starting position so your shoulders are touching the floor.

Glute-Hamstring Extensions

The glute-hamstring extension is a butt-sculpting exercise that challenges your buttocks muscles no matter how experienced you are with glute-focused training. Glute-hamstring extensions require a particular piece of equipment called a glute-hamstrings developer. To begin, lock your feet in with your quads on the main pad (not your knees or your hips). Lower your torso down until your chest is parallel to the floor and hold your body completely still for one count. Your arms can be crossed in front of your chest while you work. From here, slowly lower your torso toward the floor. As you go down, make sure to keep your chest and neck lifted and your back straight. Personally, I like to imagine I'm spreading my back up and out like Superman or a butterfly, but you can channel your own hero powers. Bring your body back up while under control, contracting in the buttocks. Use a controlled tempo during the exercise. Target a two- to three-second count on the way down and take one to two seconds to come back up. Angling your toes outward will help target the movement in your glutes versus your hamstrings. Adding weights—for example, holding dumbbells or a plate—will also up the difficulty.

If you don't have access to a glute-hamstring developer, don't give up! You can still perform a similar exercise and get similar benefits by being a bit creative. For instance, you can brace your heels under a heavy, stable object—use pads, pillows, or towels to protect your knees—to let you lean forward and lift back up. Or, even better, you can work with a partner to hold your heels as you lean forward and down. The motion might not be the same, but you can still work.

Reverse Hyperextensions

Reverse hyperextensions are a leg lift with your torso supported by a bench or apparatus—working your glutes from the opposite direction as the glute-hamstring extensions above. To perform, assume a prone position on a hyperextension machine/back extension machine/Roman chair, elevated or angled bench, or on the glute-ham raise developer. If you don't have access to more specific equipment, you can lie down on a flat bench and wrap your arms underneath it to hold your torso in place while you lift your legs. Whatever piece of equipment you choose, your legs should be angled off the end of the bench toward the floor while your torso is supported. Brace your core and straighten your legs while lifting your feet up from the floor. Flex the muscles in your hamstrings, glutes, and lower back to raise your legs from below your hip line to above the hips. Hold the top position of the movement, then lower your legs back down with control to the starting position. For more glute-building potential, adjust the angle and direction of your feet; for instance, keeping your heels together as you lift. Ankle weights, a dumbbell pressed between your feet, or bands can make this exercise even harder, as will a higher or tighter contraction at the top of the lift.

Add variety and targeted buttocks-focused work to your glute routines with glute bridges, hip thrusts, leg lifts, leg curls, and their many variations. Your glutes won't know what hit them, but you'll appreciate the results when you've finished.

JUMPS, KICKS, BURNERS, AND MORE

If you're not a fan of squats, lunges, or glute bridges, there are many other butt exercises that will shape and develop your backside. These body-weight-focused butt exercises work your booty in unique ways while strengthening your core, inner thighs, quads, and lower back. As a bonus, by recruiting muscles in your arms and upper body, with many of these movements, you'll get a total-body workout in one move. Quicken the pace to increase your heart rate and work your cardiovascular system. Push yourself to amp up those gains!

Jump Squats

Jumps squats are a phenomenal booty booster. In essence, you are jumping through a normal squat. Like a squat, you can adjust the range of movement to meet your needs and exercise focus by going deep or shallow, fast or slow. With jump squats, you add jumping height and intensity as another variable in the squat exercise. Jump squats get your heart rate up and your booty burning in a plyometric variation of the squat. Jump squats are one of the best exercises out there for creating powerful movements. As you explode up and come back down, be sure to keep your knees relaxed and land softly on your feet with your knees bent. Adding weight to the jump squat through a weighted vest, dumbbells, and the like will take your exertion—if not your jumps—into the stratosphere.

Roundhouse Kicks with Squats

You'll feel like an MMA star or kickboxing pro with this butt-sculpting exercise. From a shallow squat position, kick with your left leg to the side while punching your left arm out. Work on flexing and contracting your glutes as your leg extends. As you bring your leg back in and your foot touches the ground, go into a shallow squat. Switch sides as you work. For a bit more controlled buttocks focus, slowly lift your leg, extend it outward and then back in, turning your kick into a lateral leg extension. Use a chair or wall for support, if needed, especially to increase glute focus. Slow the move down to build the burn.

Side Leg Raise

Six different muscles work in concert to rotate your legs outward from the hip. The side leg raise lights a fire under the sides of your rear, hips, and outer thighs. To perform side leg rises, lie on your left side with your left arm flat overhead on the floor or bent under your head for support, and your head propped up on your left bicep or hand. Place your right hand on the floor in front of you to balance and brace yourself. With both feet flexed, lift your right leg up to about a 45-degree angle—about 2 to 3 feet off floor. Hold briefly at the top before slowly lowering your leg back down. Repeat for your targeted reps (e.g., 8 to 12) and then switch sides. To make the exercise easier, bend your knees and keep your feet together, only lifting your top knee up and down. The move will resemble a clam shell opening, which is what this variation of the exercise is called. (See the clam below for more details.) To make the exercise more challenging, add ankle weights or exercise bands.

The Clam

From your side with your thigh and hip on the floor and your torso supported by your arm with your forearm on the ground, bend your knees and let your legs rest one on top of the other. Maintaining bent knees, lift your top leg, bringing your knee away from the supporting leg while keeping the soles of your feet together. Your legs will open and close like a clam. This Pilates move sounds gentle, but a few reps can do a number on your glutes and inner thighs. For an added challenge, place a looped resistance band above your knees around your thighs.

Landmine Kickback / Donkey Kick

The landmine donkey kick is a true glute killer. This move hits both the working leg and the stabilizing one. To perform, use a landmine or a barbell braced against something stable. Support the end of the barbell in the bend behind your knee on your working leg. Leaning forward for stability, lift and kick back in a smooth controlled motion. The end of the barbell will move up and back and your glutes will fire. Rest your hand or hands on something stable like a bench or wall to help keep your balance and to let you lift more weight. Add more weight and greater distance of leg travel for more challenge and gains.

Standing Hydrant

The standing hydrant is an essential barre exercise that can easily be converted to a butt-blasting booty builder. The standing hydrant strengthens the core, hip flexors, and all parts of the glutes. To begin, stand upright with good posture, your feet shoulder-width apart, and your hands on your hips. Lift your left leg up and out to the side with your knee bent (channel your inner pup marking its territory if you like). Stop the lift and hold momentarily when your thigh is parallel to the floor—your knee will be even with your hip. Slowly bring your left foot back to the floor. Repeat for your targeted reps (e.g., 8 to 12) and then switch sides. To make the exercise easier, don't lift your thigh up all the way to parallel with the floor; instead, lift the knee about halfway up. To make the exercise more challenging, add ankle weights or exercise bands or lift your leg higher and feel the burn!

· · ·

Treadmill Skate

If you thought treadmills were only meant for running, you were wrong. The treadmill skate uses the movement of a treadmill to help you kick one leg back and crunch your glutes. To do the treadmill skate, stand with one leg on the stationary edge of the treadmill while your hands hold onto the treadmill arms for stability. As the treadmill moves beneath you, bring your exercising leg forward and back in an exaggerated run, barely brushing the moving surface as you pass your foot across the deck of the treadmill. Let the treadmill's momentum help lift your leg as you raise it behind you while actively squeezing your glutes at the end of the movement. Lower your working leg and bring it back up into the starting position. When done properly, this move looks a lot like someone kicking off on a skateboard with the rail as the board and the working leg pushing forward over the moving ground. Working one leg at a time, prepare to torch your glutes, hamstrings, and calves with this dynamic move. If you're feeling brave, you can add ankle weights or bands or greater height to raise the intensity.

Quadruped Hip Extension / Glute Kickback / Donkey Kick

While the quadruped hip extension—a single-leg lift performed from hands and knees-- may seem simple, research has shown that the glute kickback or donkey kick causes more muscle activation in the gluteus maximus and the gluteus medius when compared to many other common butt workout exercises—even squats. Plus, the flexed heel curling toward your butt activates your hamstrings nicely. Even better, this bodyweight butt move can be done anywhere. Increase the challenge with the use of resistance bands, a cable machine, ankle weights, or even a light dumbbell behind the knee.

Donkey kicks can be performed on your hands and knees or standing. For the most control and muscle focus, start on your hands and knees with your knees directly below your hips and wrists directly beneath your shoulders, while your fingers point forward. To perform the donkey kick, raise one leg up straight behind you while your hands and other leg support your body. Bend your knee slightly as you lift and press your foot up toward the sky. Avoid rotating your hips by keeping the shoulders and hips squared to the floor during the entire exercise. Feel the contraction in your glutes as you lift.

Donkey kicks target the meatiest muscle in your backside: the gluteus maximus. When you kick your leg up, tighten your lower abs to avoid sagging your hips and to protect the lower back. Adding ankle weights, bands, or a cable can really put the kick in your donkey kicks. Alternatively, keep your leg straight as you work.

Barre Kickback Pulse

Don't let the simplicity of the barre kickback pulse fool you. As you work, keep your body pitched forward from the hips so that the work is focused in the glutes and not the lower back. To perform the barre kickback pulse, stand facing the barre—if you're at home, try the back of a chair, a railing, or sturdy countertop. Place your right forearm down on the barre or other suitable support and bend both knees slightly. Keeping your knees bent, lift your outside leg out behind your body until your thigh is almost parallel to the floor. Externally rotate your hip slightly to engage the glute medius and maximus. Point your toes and place your outside hand on your hip. Lift your bent, raised leg up and down in small 1-inch pulses, keeping your hip elevated the whole time to increase the time under tension. For more challenge, add bands, ankles weights, other resistance, or increase the exercise time. To begin, try twenty pulses per leg and go from there.

Glute Kickbacks with a Cable Machine

Although mentioned as an exercise option in the kickback section above, the cable machine is worth a special callout for its booty-building potential. The cable machine is well-used and well-loved for working and developing the upper body, but this versatile piece of equipment can do a lot more than sculpt your shoulders, arms, back, and chest. In fact, the cable machine is also great for targeting all the lower-body muscle groups, not just glutes. For those used to training with free weights, the cable machine offers constant resistance while allowing you to go a little heavier. The cable machine is also great for beginners because it offers a sense of safety and control. Plus, the cable machine is chock full of variation options. In addition to offering versions of many other exercises—squats, deadlifts, lunges, bridges and more—the cable attachments allow you to work both sides, one side, or across the body to better target your areas of interest. So, get creative as you build your booty with cables!

To perform cable machine kickbacks, stand facing the cable machine and step your left foot into the handle after selecting your desired weight. Lean slightly forward and support your upper body by gently holding on to the machine. Bend your right knee slightly for support and stability and lift your left foot off the floor. Pushing through your left heel, extend your left leg as far as you can behind you without arching your back, really concentrating on contracting your glutes. Return to the starting position and repeat until you have completed all your reps for one leg before switching to the other.

Standing Abductions with Cable Machine

Standing abductions with the cable machine lets you hit your glutes from another angle, working the outsides of the glutes along with your outer thighs. To perform your standing abduction exercises, stand to the left of the cable stack with your right foot in the handle looped around your ankle. Be careful with your weight selection here, because you will not be able to lift and control as much weight lifted away from the side of your body. Bend both knees slightly and hold the machine lightly with your left arm for support. Lift your right leg as far as possible to the right side, working against the resistance of the cable, focus on concentrating the work into the sides of your glutes, and then lower the weight toward your left foot. Return to the starting position and repeat until you have completed all your reps for one leg before switching to the other.

Leg Drop and Lift

The leg drop and lift is a kickback in a plank position performed while your feet are elevated to allow more range of motion. Begin the leg drop and lift in a pushup position with your right foot on a box and your left leg extended parallel to the floor with your foot flexed. Drop the elevated left leg down to your torso just above the floor. Then, lift your left leg back up behind you while flexing your glutes until your hip and shoulders are aligned. Immediately drop your left toes back to the floor and repeat the lift. Add variation by bringing your leg beside your torso instead of underneath you before pushing your leg back up. For more difficulty, add ankle weights or bands or more height to blast your backside.

Butterfly Press or Frog Press

The butterfly or frog press starts while lying on your back. Bend your knees and bring the soles of your feet together on the floor directly in front of you. To begin, push your weight into your feet for stability as you lift your buttocks up off the ground. If you need extra support, rest your palms on the floor beside you as you push up. At the peak of the butterfly, only the sides of your feet and shoulders will be touching the ground. The butterfly or frog press may be a savasana variation in yoga, but in a strength workout, it's far from relaxing. Place the soles of your feet together and keep your knees pointed out as you pulse your booty off the floor to sculpt every angle of your glutes. Rest a dumbbell on your stomach for more booty-building activation. For an even greater challenge, combine the butterfly or frog press with a hip thrust. Elevate your back and go into a bridge like you're going to do a hip thrust, but bring your feet together in the butterfly or frog press position. Do your hip thrusts with the insides of your feet pressing together while your knees angle outward outside your hips. Your glutes will take off just like a butterfly in flight. This variation can be made even more challenging by adding weight and/or doing it with a single leg. In this further variation, your nonworking leg will be held straight in front of you while your working leg is centered with your knee angle outward, mirroring one half of the frog or butterfly press. Try angling the toes of your working leg outward to add even more glute-focused action.

Forward and Backward Bounds

Bounds are dynamic squat jumps. With this exercise, you squat down, jump forward, and then jump back. The more intensely you jump, the higher and farther you'll go. This explosive move turns up the intensity as you jump forward and back into a squat position. Use a cone, medicine ball, jump rope, weight, or any other random object as a marker for how far—or high—you need to jump. As your strength improves, you can go for additional height and distance and consider adding weights or a weighted vest. Using markers is also a good way to see how you've progressed and serves as a simple means to set distance goals.

Standing Lateral Tap

Prepare for the booty-building standing lateral tap! This exercise gives glute-boosting benefits without putting undo stress and strain on the knees. Standing lateral steps strengthen the fronts of the thighs, the outer thighs, and the side parts of your backside. To perform standing lateral taps, stand with your knees slightly bent, with your feet shoulder-width apart, your arms bent, and your fists loosely clenched or held in front of you. Begin by sliding your left leg out to the side as far as you can reach. As you extend your leg out, drive your left arm up and your right arm back. Keep your right knee slightly bent as you move. Hold your leg out momentarily at full extension before slowly drawing it back to the starting position. Repeat until you have completed all your reps for one leg before switching to the other. To make the exercise easier, keep your legs straight and lift your leg about one foot in the air instead of sliding it out. To amp up the difficulty, add exercise bands or leg weights, slow the move down, or add some explosivity to the movement.

Pretzel Side Kick

The pretzel side kick is as interesting as it is beneficial to your booty. To begin, start seated with your left knee bent directly in front of your hip and your right knee bent behind your right hip. Rotate your torso and place your hands on either side of your left knee. Brace your core as you lift your right knee and foot off the floor, keeping your chest lifted. Keep your right leg lifted and extend to kick with your leg parallel to the floor. Bend your left knee back in and release it to the floor. If lifting your knee is too challenging, start by just lifting your foot and then add the side kick when you're ready.

Front Kick

Front kicks are a great way to kick your backside into shape! Front kicks strengthen your core, your hip flexors, the fronts of your thighs, and largest muscles of your glutes. To perform front kicks, stand upright with your feet shoulder-width apart. Keep your arms bent with your fists clenched loosely in front of you. Lift your right knee to hip height and then extend your foot out. Imagine kicking something in slow motion. Drop your foot down and return your leg to the starting position. Repeat until you have completed all your reps for one leg before switching to the other. To make the exercise easier, only partially lift your knee and kick lower. To ramp up the difficulty, add exercise bands, leg weights, slow the move down, increase your kick height, and/or add some explosivity to the movement.

Box Jumps

Like bounds, box jumps are another explosive squat jump. With box jumps, you squat down, jump forward and up into the air onto a box or other supportive object, and then hop back down. The harder you jump, the higher you'll leap. Box jumps really engage your core in addition to your thighs and glutes. Not having a plyometric box is not an excuse for skipping box jumps. Any stable fixed object works. As your strength grows, push for additional height, add weights or a weighted vest, and consider incorporating other more complex movements (e.g., jumping up into the air as you drop back down and land on the ground, or other dynamic movements). Your box height is also a good way to see how you've progressed and serves as an easy way to set goals.

Depth Jumps

Depth jumps are the reverse of box jumps. Instead of jumping up onto an object, you jump or step down off the object and then jump back up into the air. Start on top of your box, ledge, or other platform. Jump or drop off the elevation and land softly on your feet with bent knees. As your feet touch the ground, absorb the impact in your legs and jump back up into the air. The harder you leap, the more muscles you'll build. As your strength grows, try additional height, add weights or a weighted vest, and consider incorporating other more complex movements (e.g., jumping up onto another box or platform in series after jumping down off the platform, or other dynamic movements).

Frog Leaps / Frog Squats

Frog leaps can be performed in multiple ways with different form. The primary goal, however, is to channel your inner frog and get that booty working! From a standing position with wide feet, sit down into a deep squat. Think of how a frog squats down with its legs folding up alongside its torso. You don't have to go that deep to start, but you can aspire to go that low. From the deep squat, leap up into the air. Depending on how you want to channel your inner frog, you can leap straight up or up and ahead. In the air, you can go straight up or raise your legs up toward your chest for added height and intensity. Lower your legs and land softly on your feet. To really mimic a frog, bring your hands down to the floor as you settle into the squat to land on all fours. The deeper you sit, the more of your hands will touch the ground (e.g., touching your fingertips, palms, or palms flat on the floor with bent elbows). Try not to lean forward as you reach down, if you reach down. Instead, squat straight down to protect your lower back. When done correctly, frog leaps are as much of a booty burner as they are a cardio scorcher. Sitting deep into a sumo squat with your butt back and down is key to getting the explosive force you need to drive up from your heels and jump high off the floor. Ribbit!

Star Jump Burpee

Whether you love or hate burpees—and I hope you love them—the star jump burpee is a great addition to a Tabata or HIIT workout. As you perform your burpees, instead of jumping straight up at the end of the movement, you'll jump into a star, extending your arms and legs out away from your body before bringing them back down below you and into the burpee. The star jump burpee may sound challenging, but you can do it! You're a star—now channel it!

Single-Leg Skip / Plyometric Skips / Bounds

If you want an alternative to plyo lunges, the single-leg skip is a great choice. From a shallow lunge position, push off your back foot, bring your leg up driving forward, and explode up into a leap. Swing your arms as you move to get extra height and to boost your heart rate. Return your elevated leg to the extended back position to repeat. When you're ready, increase the intensity by transitioning from single-leg skips to plyo or bounding skips. Exaggerate the movement and power of a normal skip to leap forward and up into the air to turn your skips into bounds that would make any track star proud.

Candlesticks

Think of candlesticks as a fun way to roll and get your booty into shape. From a standing position with your arms held straight overhead, sit straight down, bringing your bottom down to the floor right behind your feet in one smooth motion. Tuck your chin, round your back, and roll backward up onto your shoulders. Then roll forward and onto your feet as you stand straight up and jump into the air. Use your arms to help accelerate up through and into the jump. You can use the momentum of your rocking to help roll up to a standing position. The majority of the energy to get up and jump should come from your legs, glutes, and core. The compound movement is as good at sculpting your legs and backside as it is fun and beautiful.

Chair Pose with a Twist

The chair pose is a staple in yoga practice that is known for its glute-building benefits. With feet roughly shoulder-width apart, sit down part way while letting your weight settle into your heels. Be sure to breathe and hold your core firmly for stability. Raise both arms overhead to increase the difficulty. For added challenge, squat a bit lower, sinking down farther into the movement. For even more challenge, lift one leg at a time while you squat. Try to hold the position longer as you get stronger. For those wishing to take the chair pose to non-yogic insane levels, throw on a weight vest. For another variation, add a twist, and you'll also sculpt your obliques. As you sit deeper into the pose, concentrate on sinking down into your heels and sitting your butt back. With enough chair poses, your butt will have some back!

Star Jump with Horse Oblique Twist

This HIIT-meets-yoga-via-kung-fu move takes you from a star jump into a sumo squat with an oblique twist. To start, spread your legs wide in a sumo squat—or a horse stance, for you kung fu aficionados. As you reach the bottom of the squat, rotate your torso in one direction and then the other to engage your obliques. When you return to the center after rotating both ways, jump up into the air, extending your arms and legs out in a star jump. Quicken the pace to ramp up your calorie burn. For added challenge and booty building, hold dumbbells or a kettlebell in front of your chest as you squat, twist, and jump.

Donkey Kick-Through

Donkey kick-throughs are your chance to feel like a superhero or action movie star while blasting your glutes—and your whole body. To perform, squat down from a standing position and place both hands on the floor. Making sure your hands are stable and your weight is centered, kick back and up with both feet. The more comfortable and stronger you get, the higher and more controlled you'll kick, until you eventually reach a handstand. You could stop there, but this is only the first half of the kick-through. As you land with both feet and hands on the floor, sit back onto the balls of your feet and lift one arm. Kick the opposite leg out and through the space just left by your raised arm. Rotating on the balls of your feet as you bring your foot back in, raise your other arm and kick the opposite leg through the space just left by the arm. To finish, bring your leg back, put your hand back on the ground, and center yourself with both hands and feet on the ground. Kick both feet back and up into the air to begin again. Donkey kick-throughs have a great flow and look quite easy and fluid with proper execution, but don't be fooled. These are as good for your backside—and your whole body—as they are cool.

Lateral Band Walk-Out

With bands looped around your ankles, lower yourself into a partial squat. With a steady, controlled movement, walk to the side while staying in the squat position. Concentrate on pushing outward from your glutes as you move. If you don't have bands, don't worry, you can still do the lateral walks. Lateral walks target the sides of your butt— the gluteus medius— and, if done properly, will give you a serious butt lift. Side-stepping is also a critical move to get your body prepared for runs, plyometrics, WODs, or whatever adventures lie ahead.

Dolphin Kick

With your torso resting on a firm, elevated, and stable surface—one that won't move as you hang your legs over the edge—lift your legs up off the ground. The higher you lift your legs, the more your back, hips, abs, and glutes will work. Bring your legs back down and then repeat. Hold the sides of your bench or chair for stability. While this exercise works your glutes, it's also great for your back and core. For more intensity, pulse at the top of the movement before going back down, do a static hold after raising your hips and legs up towards the ceiling, or incorporate weights or bands into your kick.

Prone Frog Glute Press

The prone frog glute press is a move very similar to the dolphin kick. Unlike the dolphin kick, your legs do not remain together when you're performing the prone frog glute press. The leg lift is similar, but when you lower your legs down, you bring each leg apart, bending at the knee, and bring them under and beside you on your bench or support. To perform your prone frog glute presses, lie face down on top of a flat bench with your hips at one end of the bench. Hold the edges of your support with both hands, one on either side, keeping your spine in a neutral position. Bend your knees down 90 degrees, lowering your knees directly below your hips and just above the floor. Keeping your upper body stable and still, extend your legs back and up, touching your feet together above your body. Hold for one count, squeezing your glutes, then lower down to the starting position and repeat. To add more difficulty, add ankle weights or bands, increase your hold time, or raise your legs higher.

Seated V-Outs

Sitting on the floor is not often associated with working your whole body, but seated V-outs are one way to do just that. To do seated V-outs, sit on the floor with your legs extended out in front of you. Hold a weight like a dumbbell or kettlebell close to your chest with your elbows next to your torso. Lean back slightly and lift your legs up off the floor. Push the weight up above your head while bringing your legs out to your sides in a wide V shape, keeping your feet lifted off the floor. Lower the weight while bringing your legs together without touching the floor. Pause for a count and then repeat. To make the exercise a bit easier, perform it without the weight. To add more difficulty, add ankle weights or bands, increase the weight of the dumbbell or kettlebell, increase your hold time, or raise your legs higher off the floor.

Larson Booty Walk

A bit of fun and a bit of fantastic, the Larson booty walk is an exercise unlike any other—mostly because I made it up. If you think you or someone else made it up, that's fine, because we're building better booties together. The booty walk is just that: a walk where you concentrate on working your glutes as you move. I find this works especially well on hills. Hill walking, running, and sprinting are great for building nice legs and wonderful calves, but they are equally effective at building great glutes. You just need to be creative and listen to your body to do it.

Here's how you walk to boost that booty. Find a nice hill—and don't worry, if you live on salt flats without a change of topography in sight, you can still booty walk. Feel your muscles work as you walk. Focus on your glutes rolling and contracting with each step. Watch the muscles tighten and relax as you move. Now, accentuate that feeling. Use your buttocks as the primary impetus of your motion up the hill or across the ground. Start each step from your glutes and use them to push you up the hill or forward on flat ground. Contract your glutes through each step. This approach is similar to focusing on working your calves with every step—another great hill workout—but, since we're building better booties, we're working our glutes. The same approach works coming down the hill. Feel your glutes roll and contract with each step from the bottom to the top. Once you get the hang of it, you can booty walk anywhere!

Jumping is fun, dynamic, and brings childhood joy—not to mention some serious burn—to your booty workouts. Jump into your glute gains with plyometric exercises and novel movements.

EXERCISE VARIATIONS AND MODIFICATIONS

Glorious Glutes is filled with different exercises and approaches to develop your glutes. But one thing I need to stress is that you will ultimately have to find out what works best for you to achieve your physique goals. Whatever exercises and techniques you try, you will need to be patient, persistent, maximize your effort, listen to your body, and, above all else, be willing to push your boundaries to achieve your dreams.

Every exercise and exercise routine in *Glorious Glutes* can be modified and adapted to help you grow, develop, and push your limits. Think of yourself as a mad—or not so mad; infinitely sane, if you prefer—fitness scientist searching out the best ways to unlock your growth and development potential.

This process takes work and quite a bit of creativity.

Use this opportunity, your focused effort, your desire to improve, and your ingenuity to your advantage to help yourself develop! So, as you try out the routines, exercises, and ideas in *Glorious Glutes*, here are some variations you can use on almost any exercise to push your limits, overcome boredom and muscle adaptation, and build those buttocks!

Ways to vary almost any exercise include:

1. **Reps** – Vary the number of repetitions required to push your limits. As your strength and endurance grow, you can increase the weight you push and/or the number of repetitions performed.
2. **Sets** – Like reps, increasing or decreasing the numbers of sets for a given exercise is always an option for glutes development whether your focus is on mass or definition.
3. **Time under tension** – Vary the time working, the time spent moving through the exercise, the time held contracting the buttocks during exercise, the time lowering the weight, and/or the time relaxed at the end of the motion to reduce or extend the time of your physical exertion. You can also adjust the length and rate of time spent in the concentric (contraction) or eccentric (lengthening or extension) phases of your exercises.
4. **Weight** – Adding or subtracting weight is one of the classic ways to vary exercises. Not only can you add or subtract weight as you work through your sets, but you can also do the same within a set (e.g., drop sets or reverse drop sets). This will allow you to not only increase your total load (the amount of weight lifted in a given set) but can also extend your time under tension as you fight against muscle failure (such as when performing drop sets) to facilitate muscle growth.
5. **Explosivity / Intensity** – Adjust the amount of energy or plyometric activation you put into each exercise. For instance, explode upward and then go down slowly, accelerate through your lift starting slowly and gradually build speed as you elevate, or really exert yourself during your lift to maximize muscle engagement and get that burning pump.
6. **Join the chain—or band—gang** – Add chains or bands to your lifts to add intensity and increase resistance throughout the motion. Adding chains or bands is particularly effective in lifts involving bars like barbells but also works for dumbbells and other exercises. Bands and chains also change the amount of strength required in different portions or phases of the exercise (e.g., by adding progressive resistance and the amount of muscle engagement to the lift). Depending on how you orient

the bands and chains relative to the primary movement directions of your exercise, they can also change the angles of exertion and recruit additional muscle groups into your exercises. Bands are a particularly effective addition to many glute-focused exercises.

7. **Fly through the air with the greatest of gains** – Yes, adding jumps and explosivity to your movements can help with growth. This is a different variation, however. Adding suspension trainer work, suspending yourself at least partially in the air whether on one or both legs, can also provide novel stress and strain to your routines.

8. **Change how you move through the exercise** – Employ continuous and discontinuous movements to shock your backside. For example, include pulses at the top or bottom of your lifts while holding the weight at full muscle contraction or muscular exertion. Or include pauses or holds during the middle of the motion or at points of greatest stress or exertion. Alternatively, adjust the speed or tempo of your lifts.

9. **Exercise orientation** – Shift the orientation of your feet and the primary focus of the exercise during a movement. Classic glute-related examples include rotating your feet outward, pointing your toes in, lifting your heels off the ground, going deeper into a move, sticking your glutes farther out or tucking your buttocks in, or otherwise changing your stance during exercise.

10. **Change stress and strain direction** – Shift where the exercise tension moves through your glutes by changing where and how the exertion moves through your legs when you work. For example, pressing from your heels, toes, or the whole bottoms of your feet.

11. **Adjust the orientation of your bodyweight** – During exercise, adjust your body's angle to shift how the weight and exercise tension move through your muscles. For instance, you can lean forward, backward, sideways, adjust your shoulder and back tension, or stay centered during the exercise to increase intensity and alter the focus of exertion. Similarly, change where and how you hold your weights—beside your legs, in front of your legs,

between your legs, over your shoulders, one dumbbell in front and one behind, etc.

12. **Adjust the smoothness or continuity of your motions –** Although we tend to move fluidly through an exercise with continuity of motion, we can also change this to shock our muscles. Instead of completing the whole movement in one smooth motion, we can break it down into sections, each with different movement patterns.

13. **Surprise to overcome adaptation** – Change your routines to continue pushing your development. If your glutes have adapted to your routine, their growth will suffer. A simple way to evaluate whether your glutes have adapted to your routine is if they are no longer sore the day after you work out. If your butt isn't sore consistently, consider changing your routine or increasing your intensity during your workouts. If you haven't shocked your backside to the point of soreness, it might not respond as well as you would like with growth.

14. **Work out with a partner** – While not an exercise variation per se, working out with a partner can vary and intensify your routine, open up new exercise options, help you push harder, offer new perspectives and insights, and give you ideas for new exercises. Finding someone to exercise with can help motivate you, inspire you, and get you to the gym. When you're there, your partner can help push your limits and offer advice, particularly on issues you might otherwise miss, like poor form or whether you're pushing yourself. These opportunities coupled with your partner's encouragement can be the key to untapped gains. A partner can spot you to keep you safe, assist you so that you can lift more and longer than you thought was possible, and, most importantly, a partner can help make your workouts more fun.

15. **Create inefficiencies** – Create inefficiencies in your movements. Sometimes, good form isn't enough to get your muscles to grow. Creating inefficiencies in your exercises makes the muscles you are targeting work harder to go through the movement. Creating inefficiency is *not* advocating using bad form when you exercise. Creating inefficiencies is another way of saying, do your reps

using only—at least, as much as possible—the muscles targeted by a given lift to perform the exercise. For example, when doing lunges, your body tends to move efficiently using the least amount of effort and energy possible. While this is great for day-to-day movements, efficient motions are not necessarily the best option for muscle growth. So, when you lunge, your body's natural tendency is to engage the quads and hamstrings in addition to your glutes to facilitate the movement. However, this efficient, whole-leg movement reduces the work and potential gains your glutes receive from the exercise. Being inefficient, taking the quads and hamstrings out of the motion as much as possible, locks the glutes into the movement through strict form and encourages more muscle involvement and growth.

16. **Electrical muscle stimulation (EMS)** – Stimulating your muscles with electrical impulses can shock them into growth. Some muscles respond more effectively than others to EMS training. In the case of glutes, using EMS stimulation during your exercise routine (i.e., in conjunction with weights and intense exertion) can not only offer a novel way to train but can speed results. In this instance, EMS acts like adding additional weight and intensity to your leg routine without the risks of additional weight (e.g., muscle tears, tendon damage, joint pain, etc.). Consider EMS as another option to push yourself in new and growth-inducing ways.

17. **Blood flow restriction** – Consider wrapping your legs to restrict the blood flow to your muscles and to increase exercise intensity and difficulty.

18. **Combinations** – Any of these variations can be combined to add variety and increase effectiveness to your glute exercises.

19. **Take inspiration from your surroundings** – Use hills, water, obstacles, and structures to add variety, resistance, and challenge to your routines.

20. **Straps and other assistance** – If you're lifting heavy or are at risk of losing good form or muscle engagement, consider help. Straps, spotters, and other tools or positions to assist your lifts will allow you to focus on working the primary muscles you

want to develop (e.g., your glutes) before other muscles fail or limit your performance (e.g., your grip on heavy deadlifts).

21. **Same exercise, new equipment** – Try to improve whatever exercise or movement you're doing by adding a new piece of equipment or do it on a new piece of equipment to start. For example, do your standard barbell squats with a landmine or perform your landmine squats with a band or weight vest. Or, add glute bands to your barbell hip thrusts. Instead of squats, try a leg press. See what that shiny new piece of equipment your gym just got does and if it will help you.

22. **Be the booty** – Work on your mind-muscle connection with every rep. The more connected you are to your muscles, the more you engage and the more effectively they work and develop.

23. **Be original** – Think of your own variations and exercises to add to your exercise options.

Variety is not only the spice of life, it is also a key component of booty growth. Use these variations and modifications along with others to keep your routines fresh and your glutes growing!

Remember, this is a book about booty-building. So, although you often need to push your limits to get your backside to grow, you also need to be able to use them. Exercise intelligently and listen to your body to avoid injury. If you push yourself too hard, to the point of injury or inability to work out regularly, you won't be able to work those glutes and your goals will suffer. Use these variations to not only work smarter and more safely, but to work more effectively as well.

A WORD (OR A FEW) ON SETS AND REPS

As you exercise, a common question that comes up is how many sets and repetitions should I perform for a given exercise?

The answer depends on many factors, including your goals (e.g., muscle hypertrophy, endurance, definition, etc.), fitness level, age, muscular response to stress, overarching fitness routine, nutrition, and other factors.

However, without getting too complex, the answer can be boiled down to what works—what has worked for others and what is likely to work for you.

By exploring what works for yourself, not only do you keep an open mind and learn, but you also constantly work to overcome the plateaus—the lulls and setbacks—everyone faces while exercising and developing. Further, by adding variations to those reps—and continually challenging your muscles—you open whole worlds of possibilities beyond just worrying about sets and reps. By actively exploring and experimenting, you may also save yourself quite a bit of boredom.

In fact, one of the best ways to encourage continued muscular development is to change your sets and reps to keep your glutes—and your body as a whole—challenged.

So, instead of thinking how many reps and sets are "best", a more effective line of thinking may be to think about whether you are still challenging yourself, whether you are getting enough rest (both between sets and between exercise sessions), and whether you're working effectively when exercising. Then you can adjust the number of reps, sets, weights, exercise types, and variations accordingly.

So, while 3 sets of 8 to 12 reps of glute exercises may be a great place to start—there's a reason so many fitness professionals and researchers recommend this range, and there is some sound science behind it—this routine setup might not be what you need. Even the most optimal, science-based program won't necessarily work forever without adjustments—by you and with the program. If your gains have slowed and you're no longer seeing challenges in the gym, your muscles need new stimuli—or lack of stimuli, if you're overworking.

In bodybuilding, regardless of the body part, it's always advisable to hit a variety of rep ranges and even rest periods.

Typically, your reps will range between 5 and 30 or until failure (whether this number is low or high depends on the weight involved, your fitness, your desired goals, and fatigue).

Generally, the relationship between the number of reps and the amount of rest needed between sets is inversely proportional. However, this relationship also implies that those lower rep sets involve heavier weights which require more time to recover due to the high stress and exertion. If you're lifting light and taking extended breaks between sets, you might be hanging out instead of exercising.

Here are a few examples of different rep ranges and sets along with associated rest periods that you can use to get started for your glute exercises:

- 5 sets of 5 reps with about 120 seconds rest between sets (also known as a 5x5)
- 4 sets of 6 to 8 reps with around 100 seconds rest between sets
- 3 sets of 8-12 reps with between 75 to 90 seconds rest between sets
- 4 sets of 12-15 reps with 30 seconds rest between sets

The 5x5 scenario maximizes the mechanical tension placed on the muscles and is very useful in strength training. This approach does a great job of inducing protein synthesis and forcing neuromuscular improvements. 5x5 training is often used with more complex compound movements that engage multiple joints—think squats—for strength development. As an example, heavy weighted squats or deadlifts would be ideal for glutes 5x5 training. However, this should not stop you from experimenting with other buttocks exercises and rep ranges.

The 4 sets of 6 to 8 reps approach is one you might choose when lifting heavy to gain strength while also trying to gain mass.

The 4 sets of 12 to 15 reps approach maximizes metabolic fatigue and blood flow into the muscles to help create muscle hypertrophy—muscle growth and visible gains.

Finally, the 3 sets of 8 to 12 reps routine is an exercise classic right in the middle.

If your goal is size, you should work to stress all the various parts of the muscles' cells. Therefore, variety is crucial, not only to overcome adaptation but also to stress all muscle components. There are various ways to do this, such as spending a few weeks using one set and rep strategy at a time before switching to another, or mixing up your sets and reps in the same workout. As always, when the work becomes too easy, consider adding weight, intensity, variations, changing the time between sets, adjusting your exercise tempo, or adding more sets to keep the routine challenging.

Your glutes are like any other muscle or muscle group; the muscles in your buttocks adapt to change, challenge, and stress. Overcoming and adapting to these challenges is, after all, what allows your muscles to grow, develop, and get strong.

So, not only adjusting your sets and reps but also finding which changes are most effective for you is a science in itself.

This process does not have to be difficult, however. Make it fun! Think of exercise like play; yes, there's some suffering, but the end result and the journey to get there is totally worth it. You just need to find the right path to reach your goals. Hint: there's more than one. And don't waste any of your reps!

BE THE BOOTY

Does your booty make pancakes look thick?

I can fix that.

All you have to do is put your mind to it.

The secret to building phenomenal buttocks isn't about how much weight you can get them to move, although heavy weights and progressive overload can help. The secret to great glutes is *being the glute*, feeling the buttocks muscles work through the entire range of exertion, and then learning to make your muscles work effectively throughout the movement. Put your mind inside your muscles as you contract and relax. Put your awareness in the muscles *throughout* your exercises.

Make your muscles work with your mind *and* body.

When you put your mind into your muscles, you're not just watching, you're engaging. This attention gets you to work, not watch. And not just work, either. This attention helps you work more fully, harder than you would otherwise, and in the muscles you want to strengthen.

Use your awareness to enlist more muscle fibers, to stimulate the right muscles, to correct improper form, and to push harder and more completely than you would when just counting reps or holding a position for time.

Fully engaging in your exercises will not only focus your attention, it will also stimulate your muscles through greater activation, help you observe opportunities for advancement, show you ways to improve your form, give you ideas for ways to make your exercises more effective, and spur your muscles on to greater growth.

Glutes are no exception. Connect the mind with your muscles to get them to grow.

Use the following techniques to build your mind-muscle connection and encourage glute activation, growth, and development or come up with your own:

Weighted Glute Flexes – Stand holding dumbbells or kettlebells, or with an exercise band looped beneath your feet. Place your feet roughly shoulder-width apart. Let your arms hang loosely by your sides, as relaxed as you can. Maintaining as much relaxation throughout your body as possible, lean forward while the weights or band go down by your sides or in front of you like you're performing a Romanian deadlift. Tilt and extend your buttocks out as you lean forward. Try to keep your focus—and contraction—in your glutes as you lean. Stop going forward when the weight begins to engage your hamstrings. Lift back up slowly with your awareness fully in your glutes. Try to use only the muscles in your buttocks to lift. Concentrate on your buttocks to the point where your glutes seem like the only muscles in your body. At the top of your lift, squeeze your buttocks tightly and hold the contraction for 10 seconds. Tighten your muscles, flexing as hard as you can while supporting the weight or band as you hold. Repeat, performing 3 to 4 deadlift flexes. The more deadlift flexes you perform with full attention, the better your mind-muscle connection will be. Alternatively, perform the same routine with other glute-focused exercises concentrating on muscle engagement, activation, contraction, and flexing. For more challenge, add more weight or hold your flexed contractions for longer. Bring this same level of concentration and focus to your other buttocks exercises to fully take advantage of the movement and activate those muscles.

. . .

Flex – Yes, flex! Whenever you're standing—or sitting—in one place for extended periods, contract your butt and squeeze. Hold this position until your glutes start shaking (i.e., perform an extended isometric buttock contraction). This isometric hold is perfect for when you're sitting or standing at your desk or counter, working at a benchtop, seated at work, waiting in a meeting, or performing any other activity that has you staying in place. Flexing in place is also a great way to boost the mind-muscle connection with your glutes—and your gains! I do recommend trying to be subtle about this. When you're at work, you may not want to be on stage for more reasons than one. And please keep your face relaxed. Just because you're flexing your glutes doesn't mean you need to look like it.

Every Day is Booty Day – I mean it! Every time you work out, perform one set of exercises for glutes. You can do this set on any suitable equipment, using any glutes-focused exercise. Be creative and focus on building your mind-muscle connection as you work, so that working your buttocks —and engaging them fully—is part of your normal routine. Make what is important to you important. Focus on your dreams and make your goals part of your everyday routine so that you consistently achieve your milestones one rep and visualization at a time.

Slow Motion Squats – Do one squat. That's it! Just one. Except you're going to do your squat as slowly as possible. Try to do one squat over 60 seconds. If 60 seconds is not long enough to fully tax you, try 90 seconds or two minutes. Feel each muscle engage—and shake—as you slowly drop down and lift back up. As your strength and mind-body connection improves, extend the length of the squat. Put your mind in the muscle, focus completely, and breathe. As the pain and discomfort grow, you won't be able to do much other than focus on those burning buttocks! And this extended time under tension will become time for gains.

. . .

The mind-muscle connection is exceptionally important for muscle growth, especially with the glutes, since so many peripheral muscles are also used while working them. The mind-body connection, particularly learning to use this connection effectively, is also one of the weakest links in most people's overall fitness practice. Strengthen the mind-body link, and your booty will begin to become the ideal you dream of every day.

SUPERSET FOR SUPER GAINS

This targeted leg day routine brings together the Holy Trinity of glute exercises—the Bulgarian squat, hip thrust, and Romanian deadlift—to create a butt-building program that will blast your backside into the heavens. Depending on your glute exercise allegiances, and your thoughts on exercise Trinities, you can substitute other glute-focused movements like the barbell squat, deadlift, or reverse hyperextension into the routine.

Try this program for a month to start and consider using it as an option on your leg days going forward.

Routine:

Preparation:

Dynamic Warmup – 5 Minutes—bodyweight squats, jumping jacks, Atlas twists, bodyweight lunges, etc.
Mobility Work – 5 Minutes—leg swings, leg pulls, arm swings, etc.

· · ·

Exercises:

1. **Bulgarian Squat** – 7 reps for 3 sets. Rest one minute between sets.
   2. **Superset**:
   a. **Barbell Hip Thrusts** – 6 reps for 5 sets, and
   b. **Romanian Deadlifts** – 6 reps for 5 sets. Rest 90 to 120 seconds between supersets.
   3. **Seated Calf Raises** – 6 reps for 8 to 12 sets. Rest 30 seconds between sets.

Using heavy weights combined with a steady pace, this routine will test you every rep of the way. Be sure to prepare properly for the challenge ahead with a dynamic warm-up and mobility work to prepare your body. Moving through unweighted versions of the exercises is one way to go about this prep work. As always, use good form for all the exercises—you're not rushing to get done, you're working to get done properly so that you can benefit from your efforts. Choose relatively heavy weights that will push you with each set.

Use this program to add mass, strength, and volume to your backside. Your posterior chain will thank you, but you may need to upgrade your pants to hold the additional mass!

HIIT THOSE BUTTOCKS

High intensity training is training involving periods of exercise at or near maximal exertion followed by short periods of rest. These rest periods generally do not provide enough time for full recovery from the intense exertion of the exercise.

Tabatas, for example, are one type of HIIT training where you go through one or more intense exercises over a four-minute period. Tabatas involve eight twenty-second exertion phases broken up by eight 10-second rest phases right after exertion. So, over four minutes, you exert yourself at or near maximum effort for 20 seconds and then take a 10-second break eight times in the four-minute Tabata set.

HIIT training doesn't have to be as regimented as Tabata training. Exercises often range from 60 to 90 seconds, each performed at or near maximum exertion with rest periods ranging from a few seconds to more than the workout time.

Tabatas and HIIT can make great booty-building challenge workouts. They allow you to throw short, intense bursts of exertion at your glutes. You could, for example, mix up as many glute exercises as you can in a single HIIT session, or just focus on one.

Here are a couple of glutes-specific HIIT routines.

Consider these as idea starters as you fill in your own routines.

The options here are truly limitless. If you want to broaden these programs to work the entire leg, consider adding quadriceps, hamstring, and calf work into the rotations.

Tabata session 1:

One of our favorite HIIT sessions involves drop-set Tabatas with squats. If you don't have access to a gym with a variety of bars, weights, and cable systems, you can use bands or dumbbells at home for this routine. After warming up, for 20 seconds perform normal squats with the maximum weight you can handle—or have—for 8 to 12 reps, or as many as you can manage. Sixty to eighty percent of your one rep maximum is a good target weight to start. Follow the normal Tabata protocol of 20-second exercise phases followed by 10-second rest phases for 4 minutes. When you can no longer lift your weight with good form, drop to a lower weight during the next rest cycle and keep pushing in the following exercise phases. Drop weight as you hit failure in your sets, but only as needed—you're not trying to take the challenge out of the Tabata. If your glutes and legs are not on fire after eight successive sets with minimal rest between, you're not trying hard enough, aren't using enough weight, or aren't using good form.

Similar single-exercise Tabatas can be performed with any glute exercise of your choice. Romanian deadlifts, Bulgarian squats, hack squats, lunges, jump squats with a weight vest, Bulgarian squats, and pistol squats are some of our favorites. Many of these exercises work well at home where equipment may be more limited than at the gym.

Tabata session 2:

Another of our favorite HIIT sessions involves Tabatas with a variety of glute exercises, going through a range of different squats, lunges, kickbacks, and jumps for each exertion phase. As with HIIT session 1, if you don't have access to a gym with a variety of bars, weights, and cable systems, you can use bands or dumbbells at home. After warming up, for 20 seconds perform a glute exercise with the maximum weight you can handle—or have—for 8 to 12 reps. For each 20-second exercise period, choose a different exercise to hit those glutes from all angles with minimal rest. Any exercises presented in this book will do.

Examples you can use are single-leg pistol squats, plyometric squats, plyo split squats, deadlifts, hack squats, standard squats, lunges, kickbacks, hip thrusts, Bulgarian squats, cable leg extensions, and many more. Add variation by adjusting your foot placement, switching between single and double-leg movements, performing plyometric moves, adjusting lift tempo and movement angles, changing weight placement, adjusting movement patterns, adding pauses within the movement, and more. Adding variety to your workouts is one place where your creativity can shine.

As an alternative to these two Tabata sessions, perform equivalent HIIT routines with longer exertion and rest periods.

Note:

As you suffer through a Tabata or HIIT session, because you are working so hard, you may not be able to think as clearly and effectively as normal. As a result, you may want to plan out your exercises before you get started so you're not struggling to think of what to do next when you're exhausted and in pain and have only 10 seconds to think of what to do next and prepare for it.

Also, by planning ahead, you'll have everything you need in place to quickly switch from one exercise to the next. Ten seconds is not a long time to break between exercises. Add getting everything you need to switch from one exercise to the next into the time, and being prepared becomes critical. Adjustable dumbbells really shine here if you don't have access to a full weight rack.

HIIT training pushes you to your limits in short, intense time periods. As such, you may need significant recovery time after HIIT sessions. But, when these exercises are done right, your glutes won't know what hit them.

PARTIALS FOR PAIN—AND GROWTH

In this routine, you are going to prime your muscles for failure. After you've primed the pump for muscle growth, you'll push through the pain and work some more to blast your muscles into oblivion. This superset starts with partial reps and then moves to full range reps after you've burnt your muscle out.

You may hate me for putting you through this routine, but your glutes will thank me—after they've recovered and you're done crying on the floor.

Here's a partial rep superset routine that primes your buttocks for gains:

1. **Exercise** – Choose an exercise that you are comfortable with performing to exhaustion. Squats, deadlifts, hip thrusts, and lunges are good exercises to start because of the control and stability they allow while burning your glutes.
2. **Weight Selection and Preparation** – After warming up, choose a weight that allows you to maintain good form throughout the

exercise range. You will be performing partial reps to start, so you need to choose a weight that you can safely hold in place while you are at the point of maximum exertion in the exercise (e.g., near the middle of the rep in a squat where your legs bend at a 90-degree angle).

3. **Partial Reps** – While holding the weight(s) at the point of maximal exertion/muscular tension, perform partial reps to failure. Perform a truncated version of the exercise, moving up and down slightly above and below the point of highest tension (e.g., midway down in a squat, lunge, or deadlift). Remember, you are not performing full reps. You are priming the muscles for growth, getting them full of blood to build a pump, and prefatiguing your muscles.

4. **Full Reps** – When your legs are on fire and you cannot perform any more partial reps, *immediately* switch to normal reps over the full movement range. Aim for a target number of repetitions (e.g., 8 to 10, 10 to 12, or 15 to 20). No matter what, perform all your target reps. Your form will be terrible, your muscles will shake, and the sensations will get worse as you go on, but the blood will be flowing and your muscles will grow.

As you perform this routine, consider adding variety to keep the workout fresh, encourage engagement, avoid mental exhaustion, and continue shocking those glutes. You can change how you hold the weight (e.g., on your shoulders, in the front, or down by your sides), the amount of weight used, the type of apparatus (e.g., dumbbell, suspension bands, kettlebells, barbell, pulleys, bands, etc.), the exercise performed (e.g., squats, lunges, deadlifts, hip thrusts, jump squats, etc.), the exercise tempo, the section of the exercise performed, and any other variation to keep those gains and challenges coming.

The Partials for Pain workout is yet another way to fully fatigue your muscles, fill your buttocks with rejuvenating blood, force yourself to work through the pain and exhaustion of hard exercise, and shock your muscles into growth and development.

Remember, the path of suffering, exhaustion, and exertion leads to glorious glutes!

BUTT BLASTER ROUTINE

The butt blaster routine is a relentless assault on your backside. This routine uses a variety of exercises and workout angles that will allow you to keep powering through despite the building burn.

This routine is for 15 minutes. There are no breaks, no timeouts, and no pauses in this routine. You work as much as you can as well as you can for 15 minutes. This routine uses the "as many reps as possible" (AMRAP) approach employed in CrossFit® training. Listen to your body as you work and do the best you can without risking injury.

Workout:

Perform AMRAP for 15 minutes – continue through the exercise cycle until the time is up.

1. Frog Pumps – 20 reps.
2. Single-Leg Glute Bridges – 20 reps (10 reps on each leg).
3. Air Squats – 20 reps.
4. Lunges – 20 reps (10 reps on each leg).

Completing all the exercises sequentially is one round. Perform as many rounds as possible in 15 minutes. You have to complete all the reps of an exercise before moving to the next one.

If you want to challenge yourself and track your progress, keep score! Tally your score by counting the number of rounds you completed in the 15-minute period and note any additional reps performed on the unfinished round. Compare how you did from one workout to the next.

This is a glute-focused workout, but you will also feel the burn in your legs and hips. If you are feeling tightness or soreness in your lower back or elsewhere, check your form, slow down, or scale back on volume so that the proper areas are worked.

Consider substituting other exercises into this routine to create new challenges and to blast those buttocks!

BODYWEIGHT BUTT BUILDER ROUTINE

You don't need weights to build a better booty, especially if you're just starting your fitness journey or have lapsed in your exercise routine. This bodyweight butt builder program is proof that your mass can build a better ass.

That said, good form, patience, consistency, a healthy diet, enough sleep, adequate recovery time, squeezing and activating your glutes while working, and progressively increasing the difficulty of your routine as you get stronger and fitter will serve you well on your booty-building journey.

This bodyweight butt builder routine incorporates supersets—going from one exercise immediately to the next—along with glutecentric exercises to take your booty game to the next level.

Workout:

1. **Superset:**
    a. Glute Bridges or Hip Thrusts – 3 sets of 8 to 10 reps.
    b. Push-Ups – 3 sets of AMRAP. These can be modified to knee push-ups or partial push-ups as needed.

2. **Clamshells** – 3 sets of 10 to 12 reps per side. Rest 1 minute between sets.

3. **Superset**:

a. Superman Back Squeezes – 3 sets of 8 to 10 reps.

b. Bird Dogs or Super Dogs – 3 sets of 5 reps per side.

4. **Superset**:

a. Hamstring Leg Curls – 2 sets of 5 to 10 reps. You can use a stability ball, socks on the floor, or a towel to slide on—anything that glides or rolls that you can put your feet on to assist your leg curls.

b. Planks – 2 sets of 30- to 60-second holds.

To add more challenge—and booty-gaining potential—add weight or resistance to the exercises, increase your time under tension, change up exercises, or add more reps.

You may not thank me, but your booty will.

TWICE A WEEK GLUTE GAINS PROGRAM

There are many ways to build your booty. The following routines comprise a two-day glute workout program to build your glute muscles and improve your strength.

This program emphasizes compound, multi-joint lifts with both high eccentric (extension-based) components and concentric (contraction-based) exercises in the same session, often in higher volumes.

Due to the high exercise repetition volumes in these workouts, you may experience more muscle soreness than usual after workouts. Be sure to warm up, stretch, and cool down properly to help reduce soreness. Wait one or two rest days between sessions.

Workout 1:

1. Quadruped Banded Hip Extensions – 3 sets of 10 reps with each leg.
2. Back Squats (parallel or below) – 4 sets of 8 to 12 reps.
3. Romanian Deadlifts – 4 sets of 8 to 12 reps.
4. Single-Leg Elevated Glute Bridges – 3 sets of 10 to 12 reps.

Workout 2:

1. Banded Sumo Walk – 3 sets of 10 reps with each leg.
2. Bulgarian Split Squat – 4 sets of 8 to 12 reps with each leg.
3. Barbell Hip Thrust – 4 sets of 12 to 15 reps.
4. Side-Lying Banded Leg Raise – 3 sets of 15 to 20 reps per leg.

This twice-a-week program will hit your glutes from many angles to get them developing. Add this program to your regular exercise routine to start seeing those glutes gains!

THREE TIMES A WEEK GLUTE GAINS PROGRAM

The three times a week glutes program will—surprise, surprise—have you performing glute-focused exercises three days a week. If you're feeling brave, are already fit, or are ready for more of a challenge, you can add other leg exercises to this program or work it into your current exercise routine. This program is intended to be performed for a month, but it can be done longer or cycled on and off. Since you'll be working your buttocks three days a week, space the days out so that you have time off in between workouts.

Workout 1:

1. Barbell Hip Thrusts – 12 reps for 4 sets.
2. Banded Seated Abductions – 20 to 40 reps for 4 sets.

Workout 2:

1. Barbell Hip Thrusts – 5 reps for 4 sets.
2. Extra Range Leg Swings – 10 to 20 reps per side for 4 sets.

Workout 3:

1. Barbell Hip Thrust Isolation Hold – 60 seconds for 4 sets.
2. Banded Glute Bridge – 20 reps for 4 sets.

Here are some tips for each exercise:

Barbell Hip Thrusts – Place the barbell directly above your hips. Keep your weight in your feet and shoulder blades as you drive the weight up from your feet. Control the weight on the way down.

Banded Seated Abductions – Sit on a platform, ledge, or bench with your back straight and your feet on the floor. Loop a resistance band around your legs just above your knees. Push your knees away from each other and then slowly bring them back together, controlling the movement through each rep.

Extra Range Leg Swings – Loop an exercise band around your legs just above your knees. Place your hands and left knee on the bench in a kneeling tabletop position. Bring your working right leg forward as far as you can and then swing it back, squeezing your glutes at the top. You can use a cable machine as an alternate to a band or perform kickbacks instead. Whatever you choose, maintain good form and keep your torso straight.

Banded Glute Bridge – Loop an exercise band around your legs just above your knees. Lie on your back with your knees bent and your resting feet flat on the floor. Lift your hips up while squeezing your glutes. Do not let your knees collapse inward as you lift so that you maintain tension around all sides of your glutes.

．．．

The beauty of this three-day routine is its glute-focused simplicity. Two exercises a day to grow the booty in all ways!

FOUR TIMES A WEEK GLUTE GAINS PROGRAM

The following buttocks-focused program is a four-day glute workout designed to build mass and strength in your backside.

This program emphasizes many of the same compound lifts as the twice a week glute program. With the four days a week program, however, the daily training volume is significantly lower. This lower training volume allows your muscles to recover quicker between sessions. With faster recoveries between workouts, you can employ higher training frequencies. This higher training frequency will also let you get in more high-quality sets in a given week to help your build your booty.

Workout 1:

1. Quadruped Banded Hip Extension – 2 sets of 10 reps with each leg.
2. Back Squat (parallel or below) – 4 sets of 8 to 12 reps.
3. Single Leg Elevated Glute Bridge – 2 sets of 10 to 12 reps.

Workout 2:

1. Barbell Hip Thrust – 4 sets of 12 to 15 reps.
2. Side-Lying Banded Leg Raise – 4 sets of 12 to 15 reps with each leg.

Workout 3:

1. Front Squat – 4 sets of 8 to 10 reps.
2. Banded Clam Shell – 4 sets of 15 reps with each leg.

Workout 4:

1. Bulgarian Split Squat – 4 sets of 8 to 10 reps with each leg.
2. Cable Pull Through – 3 sets of 8 to 10 reps (heavy).
3. Banded Partial-Rep Squats – 3 sets of 45 to 60 seconds. Remain in the middle working portion/phase of the squat and target 30+ repetitions.

This program takes the mantra "every day is glute day" to heart and blasts your buttocks with high frequency, mass-building exertion. Working out four days a week, you'll never skip leg—or glute—day!

WHOLE-BODY GLUTE BUILDING PROGRAM

This whole-body program incorporates booty-building into your whole-body training regime. This way, although you'll build those glutes, you'll also work on the rest of your body too. This complete approach will build a complete body along with a better butt.

This program incorporates foundational glute-building movements—bridges, hinges, squats, and abduction—to hit your backside from every angle. Including these various exercise types into your program will work your glutes in multiple planes of movement so that your buttocks will develop and strengthen from all sides.

This four-day training program incorporates upper and lower body splits into your weekly routine, with extra glute work added to your upper body days to keep those gains coming.

This routine works each movement across a variety of rep ranges throughout the week, incorporating high volume/low intensity exercises along with high intensity/low volume exercises.

To add overload and continued challenge to the program, decrease the number of reps in reserve (RIR) for each exercise. Reps in reserve are how many more repetitions of a given exercise you can perform before complete failure. For example, 2 reps in reserve means you've chosen a weight where you could perform two more repetitions before you could not lift any more or your form has significantly deteriorated. So, if you can do 12 lunges with forty pounds before complete failure and an exercise calls for 2 reps in reserve, you would use forty pounds to do 10 repetitions. Then, the following week or weeks as your strength progresses and you work on overloading your body, you would choose a heavier weight or a higher number of reps where you have 2 reps in reserve. Alternatively, in subsequent weeks you could also drop to 1 and ultimately 0 reps in reserve.

Day 1: Monday - Lower Body

Lower body warmup, 2 rounds:

1. Spiderman Lunge with Rotation – 5 reps on each side.
2. Banded Hip Thrust – 15 reps.
3. Side Plank Rotation – 8 reps on each side.
4. Explosive Kettlebell Swing – 8 reps.

Routine:

1. Sumo Deadlifts – 4 sets of 5 reps. 3 RIR. 2 minutes rest.
2. Goblet Squat – 3 sets of 10 reps. 3 RIR. 2 minutes rest.
3. Step Back Lunges – 3 sets of 10 reps. 1 RIR. 2 minutes rest.
4. Clamshells – 3 sets of 25 reps on each side. 1 RIR. 1 minute rest.
5. Leg Extensions – 3 sets of 15 reps. 1 RIR. 1 minute rest.

Day 2: Tuesday - Upper Body

. . .

Upper body warmup, 2 rounds:

1. Cable Face Pull – 10 reps.
2. Cable Pallof Press – 8 reps per side.
3. Bent Over Chest Throw – 5 reps.

Routine:

1. Bench Press – 4 sets of 8 reps. 3 RIR. 2 minutes rest.
2. Barbell Row – 4 sets of 8 reps. 3 RIR. 2 minutes rest.
3. Dumbbell Overhead Press – 4 sets of 12 reps. 3 RIR. 2 minutes rest.
4. One-arm Dumbbell Row – 3 sets of 12 reps with each arm. 3 RIR. 1 minute rest.
5. Glute-focused Back Extensions (squeeze your glutes while working) – 3 sets of 15 reps. 1 RIR. 30 seconds rest.
6. Monster Walks – 3 sets of 30 reps. 1 RIR. 30 seconds rest.

Day 3: Thursday - Lower Body

Lower body warmup, 2 rounds:

1. One-Leg Bridge – 10 reps per side.
2. Half-Kneeling Cable Row – 8 reps on each side.
3. Side Plank + Reach – 3 sets of 5 reps on each side.

Routine:

1. Low Bar Squat – 4 sets of 8 reps. 3 RIR. 2 minutes rest.

2. Barbell Hip Thrust – 4 sets of 8 to 10 reps. 3 RIR. 2 minutes rest.
3. Bulgarian Split Squat – 4 sets of 8 reps on each side. 3 RIR. 2 minutes rest.
4. Cable Kickbacks – 3 sets of 15 reps on each side. 1 RIR. 30 seconds rest.
5. Frog Pumps – 3 sets of 30 reps. 1 RIR. 30 seconds rest.

Day 4: Friday - Upper Body

Upper body warmup, 2 rounds:

1. Feet Elevated Glute Bridge –15 reps.
2. Band Resisted Dead Bug – 8 reps on each side.
3. Banded Wall Slides – 3 reps.

Routine:

1. Barbell Z-Press – 4 sets of 8 reps. 3 RIR. 2 minutes rest.
2. T-Bar Row – 4 sets of 10 reps. 3 RIR. 2 minutes rest.
3. Half-Kneeling Dumbbell Shoulder Press – 3 sets of 10 reps on each side. 3 RIR. 1 minute rest.
4. Meadows Row – 3 sets of 10 reps on each side. 1 RIR. 1 minute rest.
5. Cable Pull Through – 3 sets of 12 reps. 1 RIR. 30 seconds rest.
6. Kettlebell Swings – 3 sets of 15 reps. 1 RIR. 30 seconds rest.
7. Seated Abductions – 3 sets of 30 reps. 1 RIR. 30 seconds rest.

With this progressive approach, you will build powerful, strong glutes while using the correct frequency and intensity for each movement. At the same time, you will train your glutes in the primary movement patterns to help your them develop. To overcome adaptation and keep those gains coming, substitute other hinging, thrusting, squatting, and abducting movements into this and other programs, increase your weight, or reduce your reps in reserve.

DOUBLE-TROUBLE WORKOUT

The double-trouble workout takes two glute-focused exercises—the deadlift and wall ball tosses—and blends them together for a routine that will test your backside and body as much as it builds it.

This is a CrossFit® style workout using as many reps as possible over 7 minutes. You will cycle between wall ball shots and deadlifts the whole time without resting or stopping. To do this routine, you will need a barbell with weights, a medicine ball, and a solid wall to throw your ball up into the air against.

Workout:

Perform AMRAP in 7 minutes.

1. Wall Ball Shots – Use a 20 or 14 lb. medicine ball to engage those glutes. Lighter balls are an option as well.
2. Deadlifts – Perform 5 deadlifts using 225 lb. or 155 lb. at the top of each minute (1:00, 2:00, 3:00, etc.)

The workout starts with you performing as many wall ball shots as you can. Then, at the top of each minute, starting at 1:00, perform 5 deadlifts. Begin the next round of wall ball shots immediately after completing the deadlifts. The weights listed are examples for men and women. Adjust the weight according to your strength and skill level.

As with other AMRAP routines, if you want to challenge yourself and track your progress, keep score! Tally your score by counting the number of rounds you completed in the seven 15-minute time periods and note any additional reps performed on the unfinished round. Compare how you did from one workout to the next to gauge your progress. For an unending range of challenges, pair other glute-focused exercises together for maximum volume, speed, and more double-trouble.

GLUTE-HAMSTRING LADDER

The glute-hamstring ladder will work your backside to the core, and work your core as well. The glute-hamstring ladder is a CrossFit® style high-volume timed workout. You will start with high reps of toes-to-bars and Romanian deadlifts and lower the number of reps sequentially as the workout progresses and you get more fatigued.

Workout (Beginner):

For time (as quickly as you can), perform a descending ladder of 10-9-8-7-6-5-4-3-2-1 reps of the following two exercises:

1. Hanging Knee Raises – Lift your knees up to your chest.
2. Romanian Deadlifts – Perform the Romanian deadlifts using 95 or 75 lbs.

Workout (Experienced):

For time (as quickly as you can), perform a descending ladder of 10-9-8-7-6-5-4-3-2-1 reps of the following two exercises:

1. Strict Toes-to-Bars – Legs as straight as possible.
2. Romanian Deadlifts – Perform the Romanian deadlifts using 135 or 115 lbs.

The weights listed are examples for men and women. Adjust the weight according to your strength and skill level. As a reminder, Romanian deadlifts begin from a standing position. Lower the weight until your hamstrings come under tension and stretch before lifting back up.

As you get fitter, your ladder times will decrease. Alternatively, if you are not concerned about time and just want a challenge, add more weight or increase the number of reps to your ladder. For variety, you can change your Romanian deadlift with another glutecentric exercise to create a new ladder.

DEADLIFT-PISTOL WORKOUT

Everybody loves a good, single-legged pistol squat. Everybody who loves glutes gains, that is. The same goes for a nice deadlift. Lifting dead weight lifts glutes like magic. The deadlift-pistol squat workout combines these two booty builders into one challenging exercise routine.

The deadlift-pistol workout is another CrossFit® style high-volume timed workout. This workout consists of three rounds, one immediately following the other. You will do all the reps of one exercise before moving on to the next. The faster you go, the sooner the pain ends! Just don't go too fast. I want your booty growing, not injured.

Workout:

Perform 21 reps for each exercise in round one, 15 reps for each exercise in round two, and finish with 9 reps for each exercise in round three.

1. Stiff-Legged Deadlifts – Pick a weight and/or random object to lift—make it interesting!

2. Left Leg Pistol Squats
3. Right Leg Pistol Squats

Time how long you took to complete the complete cycle.

Do the routine as fast as possible—no skipping exercises or reps!—and record your finishing time. Complete all 21 reps for each exercise before moving on to 15 reps and then finishing with 9 reps. As you're pushing through, remember that you are lighting a fire in your glutes to get them burning and growing!

THE WALKING DEAD(LIFT) WORKOUT

Who knew zombies had great glutes? The ones who do the walking dead(lift) workout certainly do!

Workout (Advanced):

Perform 5 rounds of the exercises below for time (as quickly as possible):

1. Deadlifts – 10 reps unbroken (that means without stopping!) with 225 or 155 lbs.
2. Single-Arm Dumbbell Overhead Walking Lunges – Walk for 50 feet holding 50 lbs. or 35 lbs. overhead.

Start a timer as soon as you start exercising. Do the exercises for 5 rounds as quickly as possible. Try to complete the 10 deadlifts without stopping (unbroken). If you rest or let go of the bar or dumbbell during the exercise, the round will not count. Rest or switch arms as needed during the overhead walking lunges.

Your score is the time on the clock when the last round of the single-arm dumbbell overhead walking lunges is completed. Faster is better, especially when running from zombies!

The weights listed are examples for men and women. Adjust the weight according to your strength and skill level. Remember, you can always add or subtract weight to make the routine easier or harder!

For an easier routine, use the following workouts instead. Don't worry, these will still get you zombie fit.

Intermediate:

Perform 5 rounds of the exercises below for time (as quickly as possible):

1. Deadlifts – 10 reps unbroken (that means without stopping!) with 135 or 95 lbs.
2. Single-Arm Dumbbell Overhead Walking Lunges – Walk for 50 feet holding 20 lbs. or 15 lbs. overhead.

Beginner:

Perform 5 rounds of the exercises below for time (as quickly as possible):

1. Deadlifts – 10 reps unbroken (that means without stopping!) with 75 or 55 lbs.
2. Walking Lunges – Walk for 50 feet holding 20 or 15 lbs. by your sides (not overhead).

If you want to be zombie fit—that is, fit enough to run away from zombies, or the hordes admiring your new and improved backside—consider the walking dead(lift) workout as preparation.

BUILD A BETTER BUTT IN THIRTY DAYS
(OR SO)

You want a better butt. Don't deny it. That's why you picked up this book. But size isn't the only thing that matters in your glutes—you're probably after a nice, tight, toned, and rounded rear, not a flat or flabby one. This butt-centered guide will help you get the glutes of your dreams in just one month (or so).

The build a better butt in 30 days program will hammer your glutes with high frequency and volume, with three days of training followed by one off day. Every training session includes at least one exercise that targets the upper glutes and one that hits the lower glutes.

Each workout session, you'll do nine moderate- to high-rep sets to optimize glute activation, metabolic stress, and time under tension, while still allowing for quick recovery so that training can resume the following day. To further boost your results, target doing one to two hours of cardio each week. Some cardio options include: incline treadmill walking, or using the elliptical, a rowing machine, or riding a stationary bike instead of running. As your strength and comfort improves, increase the amount of weight and/or reps for each exercise.

Build a Better Butt in 30 Days Program:

. . .

Do three sets of each of the three exercises per day. Increase the numbers of reps and/or weight as you progress.

Days: 1, 5, 9, 13, 17, 21, 25, 29
Banded Goblet Squat – 8 to 12 reps
Barbell Glute Bridge – 10 to 15 reps
Banded Seated Hip Abduction – 20 to 30 reps

Days: 2, 6, 10, 14, 18, 22, 26, 30
Dumbbell Reverse Lunge – 8 to 12 reps
B-stance Romanian Deadlift – 8 to 12 reps
Crouched Sumo Walk – 20 to 30 reps

Days: 3, 7, 11, 15, 19, 23, 27
Elevated Glute Bridge – 8 to 12 reps
Reverse Leg Hyper Extensions – 20 to 40 reps
Hip-hinged Abductions – 8 to 15 reps

Days: 4, 8, 12, 16, 20, 24, 28
Rest

After finishing this program, you'll be ready to put your backside front and center! Repeat as needed until you're satisfied with the results. As you start to plateau, switch to another routine or add more weight. There's no time limit on gains!

BASIC BOOTY BUILDER

The basic booty builder routine uses several key foundational glutecentric movements and builds a solid booty-enhancing routine around them. This program employs bilateral and unilateral movements to help your weak areas become strengths—and solid booties are what we're after here at *Glorious Glutes*.

In fact, your booty will be anything but basic when you're done with this booty builder.

Workout:

Squat – 4 sets of 12 reps while resting 90 seconds between sets.

  Deadlift – 4 sets of 12 reps while resting 90 seconds between sets.

  Superset:

  a. Glute Hip Raise – 4 sets of 12 reps going immediately to walking lunges with no rest between sets.

  b. Walking Lunge – 4 sets of 12 reps while resting 90 seconds between sets.

  Superset:

a. Bulgarian Split Squat – 4 sets of 12 reps going immediately to crab walks with no rest between sets.

b. Crab Walks – 4 sets of 12 reps while resting 90 seconds between sets.

To fully engage and most effectively employ all the muscles required for your lifts, activate the whole hip structure to make sure all muscles are primed for action. Exercises like the lying clam and fire hydrant can help get your hip abductors and adductors warm. Always warm up before working out, no matter how basic or advanced your booty is.

When doing this workout—and almost any other in *Glorious Glutes*—don't rely on momentum to help your lifts so you can go heavier or deeper. Control the lift through the full range of motion and go deep for those booty gains. This way, you build strength, not weakness.

This basic booty builder program combines many of the most effective glute-building exercises into a simple, straightforward routine. Don't ignore it. Your booty will thank you.

BUMP IN YOUR RUMP PROGRAM

Using compound movements (multiple joint movements that employ a variety of muscle groups) along with isolation exercises (exercises targeted on a single muscle group)—is a one-two combination perfectly suited for butt development. The bump in your rump program mixes compound and isolation exercises together in a delightful butt-building cocktail that will get your glutes growing.

This program requires two days a week to build your whole buttocks while also working your calves, quads, and hamstrings.

Workout:

Day 1: Quads/Glutes/Calves
  1. Barbell Squats or Leg Press – 4 to 5 sets of 6 to 10 reps.
  2. Leg Extensions – 3 to 4 sets of 8 to 12 reps.
  3. One Leg Rear Foot Elevated Anterior Lean Squats – 3 sets of 8 to 12 reps per leg.
  4. Superset:
  a. Two Leg Barbell Hip Thrusts or Hip Bridges – 3 sets of 10 to 15 reps.

b. Seated or Standing Calf Raises – 3 sets of 10 to 15 reps.

5. Super-Dogs – 1 set of 20 to 50 reps per side.

Day 2: Glutes/Hamstrings/Calves

1. Anterior Lunges with Dumbbells – 3 sets of 8 to 10 reps per leg.

2. Good Mornings – 3 to 4 sets of 8 to 12 reps.

3. Romanian Deadlift Variations – 2 sets of 8 to 10 reps of each RDL version.

1. Barbell or Dumbbell RDL.

2. Cable RDL – reaching down low.

3. Cable RDL – medium or high depth.

4. Superset:

a. Elevated One Leg Hip Thrusts – 3 sets of 8 to 15 reps per leg. Elevate one leg on a bench and drive up with the elevated leg. For more challenge and range of motion, elevate your torso on a second bench.

b. Seated or Standing Calf Raises – 3 sets of 10 to 15 reps.

5. Seated or Lying Hamstring Curls – 3 sets of 12 to 15 reps.

No one said building a beautiful backside would be easy, but you get out what you put in. In the case of the add bump in your rump program, you get a set of glutes to be proud of each and every day.

TWENTY-FOUR-DAY BOOTY BUILDER

The twenty-four-day booty builder plan uses a combination of strength training days that alternate between glute-focused days and hamstring-focused days. On days between the strength training sessions, you can either perform a corrective glute workout, another non-glute routine, or take the day off. The corrective workout days—and exercises—will complement the work you are doing on the other glute workout days and help to build a round, aesthetic backside by working your glutes from all angles.

The staggered structure of this program lets you lower the exercise volume on individual training days but increases the glute-building volume over the course of the three weeks—not that you necessarily need to stop after three weeks!

Program:

Glute-Focused Session - Day 1

. . .

<u>Warmup:</u>

1. Double Leg Glute Bridge – 60 seconds.
2. Single Leg Glute Bridge – 30 seconds per leg.

<u>Workout:</u>

1. Barbell Hip Thrusts – 3 to 4 sets of 10 to 12 reps. You can use dumbbells or bands if you don't have a barbell.
2. Long Leg Marches – 3 sets of 1 minute.
3. Forward Leaning Step Ups – 2 to 3 sets of 10 reps per leg.

Corrective Session – Day 2

1. Reverse Hyperextensions – 3 sets of 15 to 20 reps.
2. Hip Drops – 3 sets of 15 to 20 reps per leg. To perform, stand on an elevated block on one leg with the outer leg suspended over the floor. Slowly lower and then raise the suspended leg, lifting through your hip.

Hamstring-Focused Session – Day 3

<u>Warmup:</u>

1. Double Leg Glute Bridge – 60 seconds.

2. Single Leg Glute Bridge – 30 seconds per leg.

Workout:

1. Barbell Romanian Deadlifts – 3 to 4 sets of 10 to 12 reps.
2. Prone Hamstring Frog Curls – 3 of 1 minute.
3. Curtsy Lunges - 2 to 3 sets of 10 reps per leg.

Corrective Session – Day 4 (or off)

1. Internal Rotation Hip Lifts – 3 sets of 15 to 20 reps per leg.
2. Fire Hydrants – 3 sets of 15 to 20 reps per leg.

Glute-Focused Session Day 5

Warmup:

1. Hip Swings – 30 seconds each leg.
2. Alternating Toe Touches – 60 seconds.

Workout:

1. Single Leg Barbell Hip Thrusts – 3 to 4 sets of 8 reps per leg.

2. Dumbbell Frog Press – 3 sets of 1 minute.
3. Low Bar Squats – 3 sets of 10 to 12 reps.

1. **Corrective Session – Day 6**

1. Reverse Hyperextensions – 3 sets of 15 to 20 reps.
2. Hip Drops – 3 sets of 15 to 20 reps per leg.

Hamstring-Focused Session – Day 7

Warmup:

1. Hip Swings – 30 seconds per leg.
2. Alternating Toe Touches – 60 seconds.

Workout:

1. Dumbbell Single Leg RDLs – 3 to 4 sets of 8 reps per leg.
2. Hamstring Curls on a Slick Floor or Stability Ball – 3 sets of 1 minute.
3. Dumbbell Bulgarian Sprinters – 2 to 3 sets of 10 reps per leg.

Corrective Session - Day 8

1. Internal Rotation Hip Lifts – 3 sets of 15 to 20 reps per leg.
2. Fire Hydrants – 3 sets of 15 to 20 reps per leg.

An ideal derriere looks good from all angles. A functional backside performs well from all angles. This program will not only help you look great, but perform well too. Repeat the program as long as your gains continue from all angles.

FOUR WEEKS TO A BETTER BUTT PROGRAM

The four weeks to a better butt program will help build your bum in a month. While this routine will get you started, for truly fantastic results, you'll need to commit to a regular, long-term exercise program. This routine, and others like it elsewhere in *Glorious Glutes,* will be the key to your long-term success—and glute development.

The four weeks to a better butt program is great for home workouts because all you need are two moderately heavy to heavy weight dumbbells, a yoga mat, and a chair or bench.

You will perform each workout once or twice each week, following the number of repetitions and sets (circuits) indicated. As always, be sure to warm up before beginning. Warming up for 5 to 10 minutes by walking, jogging, performing exercises in the routine without weights or running is a good place to start. Engage your glutes as you exercise to really get your muscles firing. Push through your heels instead of your toes to really light up your glutes!

Workout One:

· · ·

Overview: Rest 30-60 seconds between each exercise. Perform 5 sets of each exercise. This routine will take about 25 minutes.

1.Dumbbell Sumo Squat – Do 10 slow reps. Push up through your heels and squeeze your glutes!

2.Regular Deadlifts with Dumbbells – Do 10 reps. Squeeze your glutes at the top for 3 to 5 seconds with each rep.

3.Weighted Step-Up with Knee Lift – Do 20 reps. Alternate your working leg with each rep.

4.Weighted Hip Thrusts – Do 10 reps. Squeeze your glutes at the top for 3 to 5 seconds with each rep.

Workout Two:

Overview: Rest 30-60 seconds between each exercise. Perform 5 sets of each exercise. This routine will take about 30 minutes.

1.Walking Lunges – Do 20 reps. Alternate your working/forward leg with each rep.

2.Single-Leg Dumbbell Deadlift – Do 10 reps per leg.

3.Dumbbell Squat – Do 10 slow reps. Go low and squeeze your glutes as you work.

4.Glute Kick-Backs – Do 10 reps per leg. Be sure to squeeze your glutes at the top.

Your results will be based on numerous factors such as your age, current fitness level, and commitment to the program. Understand that you often get out what you put in. Be dedicated, passionate, and persistent about your fitness, and the results—including the glorious glutes you're after—will come. Just keep working, keep trying, and keep evolving, just like your glutes.

THE INTERMEDIATE TO ADVANCED GLUTE BUILDER

You will not build an impressive rear through one particular exercise—at least not as efficiently and effectively as possible with a diverse program. To build the glutes of your dreams most effectively, you need to use workouts and exercises that create a significant adaptive response in your glutes and posterior chain (i.e., your hamstrings and your hip abductors, erector, and spinae). Just stringing together a series of exercises and workouts won't do—or not as well as you may want.

For best results, you need to address and overcome any limitations that might be holding back your growth and development (e.g., consistency in training, lapses in mental focus, mobility limitations, coordination problems, limited range of movement, lack of progressive resistance and adaptive response, etc.). This glute builder program is designed to help overcome these shortcomings and build a better backside.

This glute builder routine is designed for intermediate and advanced exercisers. Perform each workout twice a week for 3 weeks on nonconsecutive days with two days between sessions (e.g., exercise on Monday and Thursday, or on Tuesday and Friday).

Workout:

. . .

Weeks 1 to 3

1. Safety Bar Split Squat – 4 sets of 10 to 12 reps per leg while resting 2 to 3 minutes between sets.
2. Sumo Deadlift with Hip Extension – 3 sets of 8 to 10 reps while resting 2 to 3 minutes between sets. Be sure to squeeze your glutes at the top of the deadlift.
3. Barbell Back Squat – 3 sets of 10 to 12 reps while resting 2 to 3 minutes between sets. Be sure to get your thighs below parallel.
4. Forty-Five Degree Lower Back Extension – 3 sets of 15 to 20 reps while resting 1 minute between sets. Be sure to keep your knees locked, flex and extend in your lumbar spine, and do an isometric squeeze for 2 seconds at the top of the movement.

Weeks 4 to 6

1. Forward Lunge with Barbell – 4 sets of 6 to 8 reps per leg while resting 15 seconds between sets.
2. Podium Trap Bar Deadlift – 4 sets of 8 to 10 reps while resting 3 to 4 minutes between sets.
3. Wide Stance Front Squat – 3 to 4 sets of 6 to 8 reps while resting 60 to 90 seconds between sets. Be sure to drop your thighs below parallel in the lift.
4. Sled Push with full hip/leg extension – 3 to 4 sets of about 30 meters while resting 3 to 5 minutes between sets. As an alternative, if you do not have access to a sled, do: Reverse Hip Extension – 3 to 4 sets of 12 to 15 reps while resting 3 to 4 minutes between sets.

Your body—including your glutes—is a temple built one rep, one movement, at a time. Make sure you provide the best foundation possible to build on, the best plan to reach your goals, and the best path to realize your vision. This means you need to have the right mindset, effort, plan, and actions to get to your goals. This glutes builder program will help get you there, but you need to provide the work.

THE BUILD YOUR BETTER BUTT ROUTINE

I hope *Glorious Glutes* has your brain bursting with ideas to boost your butt. I also hope that *Glorious Glutes* has inspired you to you to do everything you possibly can to get your glutes to develop without giving up. Additionally, I hope that the programs and variations in *Glorious Glutes* have given you enough information to begin exploring new booty-blasting routines of your own.

However, in case you need more, I wanted to leave you with one final bonus buttocks-destroying option to keep you pushing—and glute squeezing—to your ultimate goal: glorious glutes.

This workout is simple. You make it up yourself. That's right, you make it up yourself. Choose three or four exercises presented in the exercise sections of *Glorious Glutes*. If you're brave, choose five, or throw in one you've made up yourself. Do three or four sets of these exercises. Try to choose options that complement one another to work all the muscles in your glutes from every direction. One way to do this is simply to select an exercise from each chapter on the various types of glute exercises (i.e., squats, lunges, deadlifts, bridges, and jumps/kicks).

Whatever exercises you choose, make your exercises count. Throw in variations to prevent adaptation. Continue adding weight to progressively overload your glutes to get them growing and keep getting stronger.

Concentrate, put your mind in your muscles, and really squeeze your glutes. Let the gains begin!

Workout:

1. Exercise 1 – Do 3 to 4 sets of any exercise of your choice in *Glorious Glutes* (or any glutes-related exercises I've missed). Try to choose exercises that complement one another (e.g., one from the squatting, lunging, hinging, thrusting, or kicking chapters).
2. Exercise 2 – Do 3 to 4 sets of any exercise of your choice in *Glorious Glutes* (or any glutes-related exercises I've missed). Try to choose exercises that complement one another (e.g., one from the squatting, lunging, hinging, thrusting, or kicking chapters).
3. Exercise 3 – Do 3 to 4 sets of any exercise of your choice in *Glorious Glutes* (or any glutes-related exercises I've missed). Try to choose exercises that complement one another (e.g., one from the squatting, lunging, hinging, thrusting, or kicking chapters).
4. Exercise 4 – Do 3 to 4 sets of any exercise of your choice in *Glorious Glutes* (or any glutes-related exercises I've missed). Try to choose exercises that complement one another (e.g., one from the squatting, lunging, hinging, thrusting, or kicking chapters).

As with the other routines presented in *Glorious Glutes*, the important thing about this self-guided routine is to explore, experiment, and ultimately find what works for you. Once you've found what works, keep pushing to learn and do more. The choices are limitless!

Good luck, and may the gains be with you!

STRETCHING

Stretching?

Yes, stretching!

Stretching your glutes, or any muscle for that matter, is an important key to enabling those gains you're working so hard to achieve, especially after you've exercised. When you stretch, not only do you get your blood flowing to help your muscles heal and grow, but also you ensure that you'll be able to use them over a full range of motion, and, most importantly, you'll be able to make the most of those gains throughout the rest of your life.

Here are a few nice glutes stretches to get you prepared to blast those buns, build your backside, help your butt recover, and get yourself living the best life possible—showing off that new and improved booty!

1. **Lying Pigeon or Figure-Four** – Start on your hands and knees. Pull your left knee toward the outside of your left wrist. Keeping your shin on the floor, rotate your left ankle towards your right wrist so your shin stretches out perpendicular to your body. If holding your knee close to a 90-degree angle is too much, keep your knee bent. Slide your right leg back so it extends out fully

behind you. Keep your hips squared and allow your upper body to fold forward. Let your weight draw you deeper into the stretch. Breathe and relax into the stretch for 5 to 10 long breaths. Repeat on the other side. If the sensation is too intense, place a yoga block or folded blanket beneath your hips, don't go as deeply into the stretch, don't lean forward, try adjusting the angle of your knee, or try the elevated pigeon below instead. Note: pigeon stretches are also sometimes called figure-four stretches and have multiple names and variations in yoga.

2. **Elevated Pigeon** – Stand as close to a table, box, ledge, or your bed as you can. Lift your left leg up with your knee bent so your leg forms a 90-degree angle, and rest your knee and ankle on the bed or table in front of you so your knee and ankle rest parallel to its edge in front of you. Hinge forward towards your shin as much as is comfortable, releasing into the stretch with each exhale. Adjust your position to feel the stretch in your glutes. After a few rounds of breath, switch sides and repeat.

3. **Lying Figure-Four Stretch** – Lie on your back with your knees bent and your feet on the floor. Cross your left ankle over your right knee. Pull your right knee towards you so your right foot lifts up off the floor. Use your hands to pull your right thigh towards you. Hold for 30 to 60 seconds before repeating on the other side. The lying figure-four is an excellent glute stretch. Pulling your leg closer to your body will really concentrate the stretch across your gluteus muscles.

4. **Seated Figure-Four Stretch** – Sometimes called the seated pigeon, the seated figure-four stretch helps to loosen up your glutes and surrounding muscles. To begin, sit upright in a sturdy chair or on a stability ball. Place your right ankle on your left thigh just above your knee. Place your hands on your shins. Keeping your spine straight, lean slightly forward to deepen the stretch. Hold for 20 to 30 seconds. Return to the starting position when done. Repeat with the other leg. In addition to chair and stability ball stretches, you can also stretch your glutes similarly by sitting on the ground or standing.

5. **Standing Pigeon / Figure-Four Stretch** – This move is the

standing version of the seated figure-four stretch. It's an effective way of relieving tightness in your glutes, hips, and back. To begin, stand up straight. Cross your left ankle over your right thigh just above the knee to make your legs form the shape of the number 4. Hold on to a chair, desk, or wall for support if needed. Slowly bend your right knee, moving your hips down into a seated squat position. Pause when you feel a stretch in your left glute. Hold for 20 to 30 seconds. When finished, return to the starting position. Repeat with the other leg.

6. **Lateral Hip Stretch** – Lie on the floor with your legs bent and your feet flat on the floor with your arms extended out to the sides at shoulder height. With stacked knees and rotating from the hips, drop both knees to one side and look over your opposite shoulder. Hold the stretch for up to 2 minutes total. Switch sides and repeat. For added intensity, straighten out the lower leg while keeping the top leg bent. You can also press downward on the bent top leg to add further engagement in the stretch in your hips and lower back.

7. **Lying Cross-Body Stretch / Knee Hug** – Lie on your back with both legs outstretched. Bend your left knee in towards your chest and use your hands to pull the knee diagonally across your torso towards your right shoulder. Keeping your back flat on the floor, continue to pull the knee as close to your right shoulder as you can comfortably. Hold the stretch for up to two minutes total. Switch sides and repeat.

8. **Reclining Knee to Chest** – Start by lying on your back with your legs straight out in front of you. Bend your left knee and wrap your arms around your shin as you gently pull your knee up to your chest. This stretch is similar to the lying cross-body hug above, except you pull your stretching leg straight up and back instead of diagonally across your body. You can easily transition between the reclining knee to chest and lying cross-body stretch to work your glutes and upper legs from multiple angles.

9. **Yogi Squat Pose** – Stand with your feet wider than hip-width distance apart, with your toes facing either straight ahead or slightly outwards—like you're doing a deep sumo squat. Bend

your knees and squat down as far as possible so that your hips come below your knees. Try to keep your back as straight and upright as possible. Pressing your hands together and your elbows against the insides of your knees will help with stability and also work to open your hips as you stretch. Hold for at least five rounds of deep breaths.

10. **Standing Straddle** – Stand with your feet two to three feet apart with your toes angled forward or slightly inward. Hinge from the hips to fold forward at the waist and bend toward the ground. For further intensity in the stretch, move your hands and torso toward each leg individually, grab your ankles to pull down, or reach back and behind between your legs. Walk your hands to your right ankle and reach as far down as you can. Hold for one to two minutes before walking your hands to your left ankle. That's one rep.

11. **Child's Pose** – Start on your hands and knees, with your knees planted out wider than your hips. Sit back onto your heels so your stomach lowers between your thighs and reach your arms and upper body forward. Keep your torso long as you continue to press your hips back and reach your arms out. If comfortable, rest your forehead on the floor. Hold the position for as many rounds of breath as desired.

12. **Kneeling Lunge Stretch** – Lower down into a kneeling lunge with your right knee on the ground and your left foot planted in front of you. Place your hands on your hips and gently push your left hip towards your left foot. Maintain stability with a tight core. Hold the position for a few rounds of breaths, switch sides, and repeat. Straighten out your back leg and lean forward for additional intensity in the stretch. Place your hands or elbows on the ground for additional support and stretch as needed.

13. **Rotated Low Lunge** – Start in a high plank position with your hands directly under your shoulders. Bend your left knee to bring your left foot outside of your left hand, ensuring your left knee is in line with your left ankle. Lift your left arm toward the ceiling, rotating your chest towards your left knee. Look over

your left shoulder toward the ceiling. Your body should form a straight line from your head to your right heel. Hold for one to two minutes before repeating the movement on the opposite side. That's one rep. To simplify the stretch, do not rotate your body or lift your arm toward the ceiling.

14. **90/90** – To perform the 90/90 stretch, sit on the floor with your legs straight out in front of you. Bend your right knee 90 degrees so that your shin is parallel with your hips while your leg remains out in front of your body. At the same time, swing your left leg around to the left side so you can bend your left knee 90 degrees, keeping your knee directly in line with your hip. Flex both feet, sit tall, and gently press your fingertips into the floor for balance. For a deeper stretch, hinge at the hips and slowly lean forward, directing your belly button toward your right calf. Hold for one to two minutes before repeating the movement on the other side. That's one rep.

15. **Seated Glute Stretch** – Start seated on the floor and extend your legs out in front of you. Keeping your back straight, lift your left leg and place your left ankle on your right knee. Lean slightly forward to deepen the stretch. Hold for 20 to 60 seconds, then repeat on the opposite side. This simple stretch helps relieve tightness in your glutes, hips, and back. If your hips need more support, sit on a yoga block or folded towel.

16. **Downward-Facing Dog** – Downward-facing dog is a traditional yoga pose. It stretches many muscles, including your upper body, hamstrings, calves, and glutes. Start in a pushup / plank position with your hands shoulder-width apart and your legs together. Straighten your body and engage your core. Move your hips back and up, forming an upside-down V with your body. Straighten your arms and place your head between your shoulders, keeping your head in line with your spine. Reach your heels toward the floor. Hold for 20 to 60 seconds. Return to the starting position by hinging at your hips and shoulders back down into a plank. To ease the stretch and provide extra wrist support, you can place each hand on a yoga block. Bend your knees if you need to reduce the stretch intensity. This may help

straighten your back, ensuring that your body stays in an upside-down V shape.

17. **Seated Twist / Pretzel** – To begin, sit on the ground and stretch your legs out in front of you. Place your left arm behind you and bring your left leg over the right, placing your left foot on the floor near your right knee. Position your right arm over your left knee with your palm facing outward. Twist to the left and use your right arm to pull your left knee inward. Hold this position for 20 to 60 seconds. Untwist and repeat on the other side. This is also a great stretch for your lower back.

18. **Piriformis Foam Rolling** – Sit on a foam roller and lean to the right side so that only your right glute rests on the roller. Roll back and forth over each sore or tight spot for about 30 seconds. Find any hot spots and settle into them, breathing and relaxing until the muscle loosens. Spend as long as needed on one side in each tight area before switching and repeating on the other side.

19. **Lateral / Forward and Backward Hip or Leg Swings** – Stand facing a stable surface (like a table, chair, or wall) that allows you to stand tall. With both hands on this surface, lift your right leg out to your right and swing it laterally to the left so that your leg crosses the front of your body as if your leg is performing a golf swing. Continue for 10 to 20 repetitions, swinging your leg higher and higher in each direction as your glute muscles relax. Switch sides and repeat. A similar stretch can be performed by swinging your leg forward and backward instead of side to side.

Almost any stretch that works for your legs can be shifted into a glute stretch with a little modification of your foot, torso, and hip positions. All you have to do is move your body slightly until you feel the stretch in the right muscles.

Play with angles to find the best stretches for you.

Now that you've worked those muscles out, go stretch, recover, and get some rest. You'll be well on your way to building a better booty when you're done.

WHAT'S NEXT?

What's next?

The honest answer to that question is up to you. Just as you determine how hard you work and how much success you have in life, you will also determine how much your glutes grow and how well they are maintained.

Personally, I exercise my legs and glutes once or twice a week through a dedicated routine—not including other days where they're worked as a secondary muscle group, like when I'm doing cardio. This is the level of commitment required for me to see results. Since I started working with this level of dedication, my booty has blossomed.

Since I am a hard gainer and don't maintain muscle mass easily, I know that if I stop exercising hard, varying my routines, and challenging myself, I will not see additional growth and development. I also know that if I do not work to maintain what I have gained, this progress will gradually disappear. With any luck, the road to your goals will be easier than mine (hopefully, much easier). But whatever your journey, *Glorious Glutes* will help get you there.

So, the choice is yours. I believe *Glorious Glutes* offers you the tools needed to help you achieve the backside of your dreams, and I hope the ideas I've presented have inspired you to push and strive for your goals.

Remember, your glutes, like your life, are what you make of them.

I want you to keep pushing, to never stop exploring, and to continually develop.

Then your glutes won't be the only things that are glorious.

Here's to being glorious!

—Rhys Larson

HELP SPREAD THE WORD!

Thank you for taking the time to pick up and read this exercise guide. I hope you found *Beastly Body* worthwhile and that you'll crush your fitness goals as a result.

If you appreciated this book, please help spread the word and consider leaving a review.

Everyone needs a beastly body.

Together, with hard work and dedication, we can make that possible.

Many thanks, and many gains!

—Rhys Larson

The publisher and the author strongly recommend that you consult with your physician and follow their advice before beginning any exercise program. Before starting, you should be in good physical condition and be able to participate in exercise programs, physical activities, and physical and mental exertion. The author is not a licensed healthcare provider and represents that they have no expertise in diagnosing, examining, or treating medical conditions of any kind, or in determining the effects of any specific exercise on a medical condition.

You should understand that when participating in any exercise or exercise program, there is the possibility of physical injury. If you engage in these exercises or exercise programs, you agree that you do so at your own risk, are voluntarily participating in these activities, assume all risk of injury to yourself, and agree to release and discharge the publisher and the author from any and all claims or causes of action, known or unknown, arising out of the contents of this book.

The publisher and the author advise you to take full responsibility for your safety, physical and mental health, and know your limits. Before practicing the skills, exercises, and activities described in this book, be sure that your equipment is well-maintained and you do not take risks beyond your level of experience, aptitude, training, and comfort.

The publisher and author of this book very much hope you achieve your training goals. However, this book and the programs contained in it are no guarantee of success. Knowledge, training techniques, and exercise approaches change over time. Ultimately, you must find out what works best for you to achieve your goals. I hope you succeed.

Thank you and enjoy!

Made in the USA
Las Vegas, NV
27 December 2024